Alcohol Education

Alcohol Education

What We Must Do

David J. Hanson

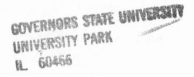
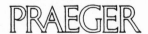

Westport, Connecticut
London

Library of Congress Cataloging-in-Publication Data

Hanson, David J., 1941–
    Alcohol education : what we must do / David J. Hanson.
      p.   cm.
    Includes bibliographical references and indexes.
    ISBN 0–275–95561–3 (alk. paper)
    1. Alcoholism—Study and teaching—United States. I. Title.
    HV5128.U5H35 1996
    362.29′2′071073—dc20   96–15325

British Library Cataloguing in Publication Data is available.

Library of Congress Catalog Card Number: 96–15325
ISBN: 0–275–95561–3

First published in 1996

Praeger Publishers, 88 Post Road West, Westport, CT 06881
An imprint of Greenwood Publishing Group, Inc.

Printed in the United States of America

The paper used in this book complies with the
Permanent Paper Standard issued by the National
Information Standards Organization (Z39.48–1984).

10 9 8 7 6 5 4 3 2 1

To

Archie and Louise

and to

the memory of my parents

Contents

Acknowledgments

The publication of any book requires the assistance of many people. Kathy LaClair and Holly Chambers of the library at the State University of New York College at Potsdam provided invaluable help and Deborah Ross and Marcia Goldstein of Praeger were especially helpful.

Guiding the book from the first drafts, through numerous revisions, to the final copy was Jackie Rush. Her hard work, accuracy, attention to detail, seemingly infinite patience, and good humor greatly facilitated the entire effort.

Introduction

Beverage alcohol has been praised as a sign of refinement, a social lubricant, a source of relaxation, an enchancer of food, a healthful tonic, and a complement to celebration and good times. But it has also been cursed as a poison, a cause of crime, a defiler of innocence, a destroyer of happy families, and a cause of disease and death. People in the United States tend to have strong, and often mixed, feelings about beverage alcohol. This has long been the case. For this reason, public policy toward it has changed repeatedly as successive waves of various prohibitionist and neo-prohibitionist movements have ebbed and flowed across the country.

One of these movements led to the widespread establishment of alcohol education programs over 100 year ago. Current alcohol education reflects both its abstinence origins at that time as well as the dramatic expansion of drug education several decades ago.

In spite of noble intentions and the expenditure of massive amounts of time, energy, and money the best evidence shows that current abstinence-oriented alcohol education is ineffective. Simply doing more of what is not working will not lead to success; it is essential that we re-think our approach to the problem. Our youth are too important and the stakes are too high to do otherwise.

Several recommendations for change are presented in the final chapter of this book. The research has proven that we must promote the development and evaluation of diverse responsible alcohol use curricula based on a sociocultural understanding of how best to reduce alcohol abuse.

1

Americans
and
Alcohol

Alcohol has always been an important part of American life, but the way Americans view alcohol has changed over time. In the Colonial period (1492–1775) alcohol was seen as the "good creature of God" but with the social and economic upheavals associated with the Revolution it was often blamed as the cause of those problems. Some began to call for the temperate or moderate use of alcohol, and with the passage of time temperance advocates promoted voluntary abstinence. Increasingly frustrated, these advocates soon insisted that no one should be permitted to drink in any quantity. The "good creature of God" became Demon Rum. Following the Civil War, the so-called temperance movement became a cause actively promoted by a growing women's movement and most Protestant churches. The Women's Christian Temperance Union (WCTU) crusaded for mandatory alcohol education and developed a virtual monopoly over the content of that instruction. A confluence of events led to the adoption of national prohibition at the beginning of World War I, but the noble experiment soon proved to be a failure. Instead of delivering the nation from poverty, crime and other problems it brought about even more serious problems and was overwhelmingly rejected and subsequently repealed. However, the prohibitionist impulse never died. While it was largely dormant for decades, it would later re-emerge in a new guise.

THE EARLY YEARS

As the Puritans loaded provisions onto the *Mayflower* before casting off for the New World, they brought on board more beer than water (Royce, 1981, p. 38). This reflected their[1] traditional drinking beliefs, attitudes, and behaviors—they saw alcohol as a natural and normal part of life. Their religious tradition taught them that alcohol was created by God and inherently good. Jesus had used wine and approved of its moderate consumption.[2] Their experience showed them that it was

Some material in this chapter has been adapted and revised from Hanson (1995a).

safer to drink alcohol than the typically polluted water. Alcohol was also an effective analgesic, provided energy necessary for hard work, and generally enhanced the quality of life. Alcohol was also thought to serve as a social lubricant, provide entertainment, facilitate relaxation, contribute to the enjoyment of food, and provide pharmacological pleasure.

For hundreds of years their English ancestors had enjoyed beer and ale. Both in England and in the New World, people of both sexes and all ages typically drank beer with their meals. Because importing a continuing supply of beer was expensive, the early settlers brewed their own. However, it was difficult to make the beer they were accustomed to because wild yeasts caused problems in fermentation and resulted in a bitter, unappetizing brew (Rorabaugh, 1993, p. 2135).

But these early adventurers did not give up. While wild hops grew in New England, hop seeds were ordered from England in order to cultivate an adequate supply for traditional beer. In the meantime, the colonists improvised a beer made from red and black spruce twigs boiled in water, as well as a ginger beer. A poem from the 1630s reflected their determination and ingenuity:

> If barley be wanting to make into malt,
> We must be content and think it no fault,
> For we can make liquor to sweeten our lips,
> Of pumpkins, and parsnips, and walnut-tree chips.
> (Lender and Martin, 1982, p. 5)

As intricacies of brewing in the New World were mastered, beers became widely available and "many farmers made their own with the help of a malster who malted their barley, or more often, corn" (Mendelson and Mello, 1985, p. 9). A brewery was one of Harvard College's first construction projects so that a steady supply of beer could be served in the student dining halls (Furnas, 1965, p. 20), and Connecticut required each town to ensure that a place could be made available for the purchase of beer and ale (Krout, 1925, p. 7).

Beer was designated X, XX, or XXX according to its alcohol content. The weakest and most commonly available beer was made by soaking grain in water. But this "small beer" spoiled quickly because of its low alcohol content and had to be consumed quickly. Brewing beer was the homemaker's responsibility and was done once or twice a week. "Ships beers" were stronger and also readily available. But the strongest beer, brewed with malt and extra sugar, was expensive and uncommon. (Rorabaugh, 1993, p. 2135; Mendelson and Mello, 1985, p. 9).

The colonists also learned to make a wide variety of wine from fruits, including strawberries, cranberries, blackberries, elderberries, gooseberries, and currants. They made wines from numerous vegetables, including carrots, tomatoes, onions, beets, celery, squash, corn silk, dandelions, and goldenrod. They additionally made wine from such products as flowers, herbs, and even oak leaves (Mendelson and Mello, 1985, p. 9). Early on, French vine-growers were brought to the New World to teach settlers how to cultivate grapes (Krout, 1925, p. 32).

Cider had been popular in England but apples were not native to New England. The first orchard, grown from English seed, was planted promptly, and over time apples became abundant in the colonies. Apple juice was typically fermented in barrels over the winter (Schlaadt, 1992, pp. 5, 8). Sometimes honey or cane sugar was added, increasing the alcohol content and creating natural carbonation—"apple champagne" was a special treat. "Cider was served to every member of the family at breakfast, dinner, and supper. Cider was consumed in the fields between meals, and was a regular staple at all the communal social functions" (Mendelson and Mello, 1985, p. 9).

Colonists adhered to the traditional belief that distilled spirits were *aqua vitae*, or water of life (Furnas, 1965, p. 18). However, rum was not commonly available until after 1650, when it was imported from the Caribbean. The cost of rum dropped after the colonists began importing molasses and cane sugar directly and distilled their own. By 1657, a rum distillery was operating in Boston. It was highly successful and within a generation the production of rum became colonial New England's largest and most prosperous industry (Roueché, 1963, p. 178).

In the profitable "Triangle Trade," rum was traded for West African slaves, who were then traded to the West Indians for more molasses to be made into more rum. This three point trading arrangement became a very important part of colonial commercial life and prosperity (Schlaadt, 1992, pp. 8–9). Almost every important town from Massachusetts to the Carolinas had a rum distillery to meet the local demand, which had increased dramatically. Rum was often enjoyed in mixed drinks, including flip. This was a popular winter beverage made of rum and beer sweetened with sugar and warmed by plunging a red-hot fireplace poker into the serving mug (Mendelson and Mello, 1985, p. 10).

MODERATION WAS THE NORM

Alcohol was viewed positively while its *abuse* was condemned. "In 1673, Increase Mather praised alcohol, saying that 'Drink is in itself a creature of God, and to be received with thankfulness'" (Mendelson and Mello, 1985, p. 10). Consistent with that belief, toddlers drank beer, wine, and cider with their parents and regular use was seen as healthful for everyone (Asbury, 1968, pp. 3–4; Sinclair, 1962, pp. 36–37; Popham, 1978, pp. 267–277). For more than 30 years, because of this belief, abstainers had to pay one life insurance company rates 10 percent higher than that for drinkers. This was because the abstainer was considered "thin and watery, and as mentally cranked, in that he repudiated the good creatures of God as found in alcoholic drinks" (Kobler, 1973, p. 26).

A historian has pointed out that:

Alcohol was pervasive in American society; it crossed regional, sexual, racial, and class lines. Americans drank at home and abroad, alone and together, at work and at play, in fun and in earnest. They drank from the crack of dawn to the crack of dawn. At nights taverns were filled with boisterous, mirth-making tipplers. Americans drank before meals, with meals, and after meals. They drank while working in the fields and while travelling across half a continent. They drank in their youth, and, if they lived long enough, in their old age. They drank at formal events, such as weddings, ministerial ordinations, and wakes, and on no occasion—by the fireside of an evening, on a hot afternoon, when the mood called. From sophisticated Andover to frontier Illinois, from Ohio to Georgia, in lumbercamps and on satin settees, in log taverns and at fashionable New York hotels, the American greeting was, "Come, Sir, take a dram first." Seldom was it refused. (Rorabaugh, 1979, pp. 20–21)

SOCIAL CONTROLS WERE STRONG

In colonial America, informal social controls helped maintain the expectation that the abuse of alcohol was unacceptable. There was a clear consensus that while alcohol was a gift from God its abuse was from the Devil. "Drunkenness was condemned and punished, but only as an abuse of a God-given gift. Drink itself was not looked upon as culpable, any more than food deserved blame for the sin of gluttony. Excess was a personal indiscretion" (Aaron and Musto, 1981, p. 132).

Informal social controls operated both in the home and in the larger community:

Central to the drinking culture of colonial life was the tavern (used here as a term to cover inns, taverns, and ordinaries—any licensed establishment where alcohol was served on the premises). The role of the tavern in colonial America and the attitudes toward it were quite different from what they would become in the nineteenth century. The tavern was considered an integral part of community life, second only in importance to the meetinghouse, which served as the church, town hall, and courtroom. The laws of most colonies required towns to license suitable persons to sell wine and spirits for the convenience of travelers and town dwellers; failure to do so could result in a fine. Contrary to the modern practice of keeping alcohol outlets a certain distance from schools and churches, colonial taverns were often required to be located near the meetinghouse or church. In towns that lacked a meetinghouse or in those where the meetinghouse did not provide sufficient warmth in winter, "religious services and court sessions were held in the great room of the principal tavern; there, ecclesiastical affairs were managed, the town selectmen and county justices met to conduct the business of government, and the voters assembled for town meetings" (Popham, 1978, p. 271). Those who attended these gatherings naturally took advantage of the hospitality of the tavern, the expenses not infrequently being paid out of town funds. People also came to taverns to see plays and concerts, to attend lodge meetings, to participate in lotteries, to read newspapers, and to engage in political debate. Taverns were, in fact, more important as centers of social activity than as places in which to drink. Most drinking took place in the home or at communal gatherings. (Popham, 1978, pp. 267–277; Conroy, 1984) (Prendergast, 1987, p. 27)[3]

Tavern owners were expected not only to disperse food, drink, and hospitality, but also to monitor behavior and keep their customers in check (Aaron and Musto, 1981, pp. 132–133).

When informal controls failed, there were always legal ones. Alcohol abuse was treated with rapid and sometimes severe punishment. Habitual drinkers "were whipped or forced to wear a mark of shame. Once so labeled, they could be refused the right to purchase liquor. During the seventeenth century, all of the colonies specified a fine or prescribed the stocks for the first drunkenness offense. Repeated offenders often received sentences to hard labor or corporal punishment"

(Mendelson and Mello, 1985, p. 11; also see Krout, 1925, pp. 27–28). While infractions did occur, the general sobriety of the colonists suggests the effectiveness of their system of informal and formal controls in a population that averaged about three and a half gallons of alcohol per year per person (Rorabaugh, 1991, p. 17). That rate was dramatically higher than the present rate of consumption.

CHANGE AND REVOLUTION CREATED PROBLEMS

As the colonies grew from a rural society into a more urban one, drinking patterns began to change. Rum became increasingly popular. As the American Revolution approached, economic change and urbanization were accompanied by increasing poverty, unemployment, and crime. These emerging social problems were often blamed on drunkenness. "This simplistic scapegoating of an intoxicant . . . now seems a predictable accompaniment of social unrest and economic problems. The basic scenario has been repeated often—opium, cocaine, marijuana, alcohol, each takes its turn as demon for a day" (Mendelson and Mello, 1985, p. 15).

Following the Revolutionary War, the new nation experienced cataclysmic social, political, and economic changes that affected every segment of the new society. Social control over alcohol abuse declined, antidrunkenness ordinances were relaxed and alcohol problems increased dramatically. Drinking, which had been controlled by the tightly knit family and social fabric in the colonial period, increasingly became an individualistic activity associated with masculine aggression and antisocial behavior by the early nineteenth century (Peele, 1987, p. 69). Alcohol use became segregated by gender and age, which encouraged excessive consumption, and concern was frequently expressed over immoderate drinking. "As community life in the colonies became less cohesive and structured, the social sanctions that had kept drunkenness to a minimum began to lose their power (Schlaadt, 1992, p. 9).

The Revolution had caused a shift in the beverages consumed. When the British blockade had prevented the importation of sugar and molasses, and thereby disrupted the production of rum, a substitute was sought to meet the demand for spirits in general and for provisions for the Revolutionary Army in particular. It was found in whiskey produced largely by Scot-Irish immigrants who had settled on the frontier (Aaron and Musto, 1981, p. 135).

Even before the Revolution, whiskey had become the preferred way to use surplus grains in the frontier settlements west of the Appalachian Mountains. The expansion of a corn belt in Kentucky and Ohio had created a corn glut. There were no roads in the region and most transportation was by packhorse. It cost more to transport corn or grain than it could bring on the eastern markets, so farmers distilled it into "liquid assets" that could easily be shipped or bartered. Practically every farmer made whiskey and it became a medium of exchange (Roueché, 1960, pp. 39–40). One wrote that "Distant from a permanent market, and separate from the Eastern coasts by mountains, we have no means of bringing the product of our lands to sale either by grain or meal. We are therefore distillers by necessity, not choice" (Rorabaugh, 1979, p. 54).

By 1810, there were at least 2,000 distillers producing more than two million gallons of whiskey (Roueché, 1960, p. 42). By the 1820s, whiskey sold for twenty-five cents a gallon, making it cheaper than beer, wine, coffee, tea, or milk (Rorabaugh, 1991, p. 17). Annual consumption may have been as high as ten gallons per person (Clark, 1976, p. 20; Asbury, 1968, p. 12).[4]

This level of consumption was over four times the current rate. However, "liquor tended to be taken in small quantities throughout the day, often with meals. Instead of a morning coffee break, Americans stopped work at 11:00 a.m. to drink. A lot of work went undone but in this slow paced, preindustrial age this was not always a problem. A drunken stage coach driver posed little threat, since the horses knew the route and made their own way home" (Rorabaugh, 1991, p. 17). But not all was well. Writing at the time, the famous observer of American life, Alexis de Tocqueville, suggested that the sudden disappearance of traditional boundaries left people bereft and disoriented (Aaron and Musto, 1981, p. 136), with negative consequences for social control.

Describing the traditional mechanism that had earlier controlled drinking abuse, Aaron and Musto (1981, p. 137) have pointed out that:

Sanctions to regulate conduct, operating within an overall context of civic cohesiveness, were intended to shame the offender before the community. The stocks or the wearing of the letter "D" subjected the drunkard to ridicule, and such ceremonies of public humiliation were assumed to have a deterrent power. However, with frenzied economic and geographic mobility, exile became self-imposed. The rootless individual, seeking his fortune, living by his own wits, and answerable to no social superior, became celebrated as the national character ideal. The stable, self-policing community was demolished; the forms of behavioral management that grew out of an inherited concept of reciprocal rights and obligations became obsolete.

They (p. 137) explain that:

the combination of precipitate and bewildering change unmoored people from their sense of place, both social and physical. We do know that there was more drinking of hard liquor in settings that no longer even offered the pretense of other activities. The tavern or inn, where food and lodging provided a milieu that militated against intense drinking, gave way almost exclusively to the grogshop, essentially an early version of the saloon. Drinking became detached from earlier safeguards. And whereas before this process of detachment had provoked attempts to reassert controls, efforts at regulation became increasingly listless and ineffectual.

Solitary drinking, unencumbered by social control, increased during this time. "A sizeable number of Americans for the first time began to drink to excess by themselves. The solo binge was a new pattern of drinking in which periods of abstinence were interspersed every week, month, or season with one to three-day periods of solitary inebriation" (Rorabaugh, 1979, p. 144). "Middle- and upper-class Americans cut back their drinking drastically because it was no longer considered appropriate for an industrious life. As alcohol was eliminated from the ordinary daily routines of the middle class, when people did drink, they were more likely to go on binges where they drank all out" (Peele, 1989, p. 36).

BIRTH OF THE TEMPERANCE MOVEMENT

It was in this environment that people began seeking an explanation and a solution for drinking problems. One suggestion had come from one of the foremost physicians of the period, Dr. Benjamin Rush. In 1784, Dr. Rush published "An Inquiry into the Effects of Ardent Spirits Upon the Human Mind and Body" in which he argued that the excessive use of distilled spirits was injurious to physical and psychological health and urged abstinence from ardent spirits and moderation in the consumption of fermented beverages (Katcher, 1993, p. 275). "He envisioned a healthy American people bursting with beer, light wines, and happiness" (Asbury, 1968, p. 28).

Apparently influenced by Rush's widely distributed tract, about 200 farmers in a Connecticut community formed an association in 1789 pledging not to use distilled spirits themselves nor provide it to anyone they employed. Similar associations were formed in Virginia in 1800 and New York State in 1808. Within the next decade other temperance organizations were formed in eight states, some being statewide organizations (Asbury, 1968, pp. 28–31).

The future looked bright for the young movement, which advocated temperance or moderation rather than abstinence.[5] But many of the leaders overestimated their strength; they expanded their activities and took positions on gambling, profanation of the Sabbath, and other moral issues. They became involved in political bickering and by the early 1820s their movement stalled (Asbury, 1968, p. 31). But some stalwart leaders persevered in pressing their cause forward. The American Temperance Society was formed in 1826 and benefitted from a renewed interest in religion and morality. Within 10 years it claimed more than 8,000 local groups and over 1,500,000 members (Furnas, 1965, p. 55). By 1839, 15 temperance journals were being published (Cherrington, 1920, pp. 98–123). Simultaneously, many Protestant churches were beginning to promote temperance.

FROM TEMPERANCE TO TOTAL ABSTINENCE

Between 1830 and 1840, most temperance organizations began to argue that the only way to prevent drunkenness was to eliminate the consumption of alcohol. The Temperance Society became the Abstinence Society. The Independent Order of Good Templars, the Sons of Temperance, the Templars of Honor and Temperance, the Anti-Saloon League, the National Prohibition Party and other groups were formed and grew rapidly (Blocker, 1985, pp. 67–72). With the passage of time, "The temperance societies became more and more extreme in the measures they championed" (McConnell, 1963, p. 569). While it began by advocating the temperate or moderate use of alcohol, the movement now insisted that no one should be permitted to drink any alcohol in any quantity. And it did so with religious fervor and increasing stridency (Royce, 1981, p. 40; Sheehan, 1984b, p. 73). Even when compared to the sophisticated use of mass media today, the temperance movement still rivals the best in terms of scope, commitment, and response (Wallack, 1981, p. 211):

No effort in our era at mass communications about alcohol comes close to matching the outpouring of materials for the mass audience by the temperance movement in the nineteenth century. For decades the American public was flooded with temperance pamphlets, temperance novels, temperance newspapers, temperance sermons, and temperance lectures—the longest sustained and perhaps the largest organized effort at mass communication about a social issue that the country has ever seen. (Room, 1977, p. 22)

The prohibition of alcohol by law became a major issue in every campaign from the national and state level, to those for school board members. The issue generated deep bitterness. "It is hard for us today to grasp how profoundly this controversy pervaded every facet of American life for a century. . . . Religious and political party affiliation were so intertwined with the prohibition issue, and feelings ran so high, that it became a rule of polite society not to allow them in conversation" (Royce, 1981, pp. 40–41).

PAVING THE ROAD TO UTOPIA

A temperance leader asserted that "This [prohibition] is Christ's work . . . a holy war, and every true soldier of the Cross will fight in it" (Furnas, 1965, p. 165). Understandably, ministers were influential and important to the cause (Schmidt, 1995). They mobilized their flocks by preaching that alcohol was

the great anaconda, which wraps its coils around home altars to cripple them, to make room for Bacchus. The vampire which fans sanity to sleep while it sucks away the lifeblood. The vulture, which preys upon the vials [sic] of the nations. It defies God, despises Jesus Christ, sins against the Holy Ghost, which is sinning against light and knowledge. Above all it murders humanly. (Isaac, 1965, p. 21)

In promoting what many prohibitionists saw as their religious duty, they perfected the techniques of pressure politics (Odegard, 1928). Women in the movement even used their children as pawns to march, sing, and otherwise exert pressure at polling places. Dressed in white and clutching tiny American flags, the children would await their order to descend upon an unsuspecting "wet" as he approached the voting booth.

The Anti-Saloon League stressed its religious character and since it acted as an agent of the churches and therefore was working for God, anything it did was seen as moral and justified because it was working to bring about the Lord's will:

It didn't necessarily include the outright purchase of a politician, nor did it preclude such a buy if the situation warranted. In general, however, and briefly, it consisted in swarming into a contested area and bringing every imaginable sort of pressure to bear upon the candidates and officeholders; in saturating the country with speakers and literature; in laying down a barrage of abuse, insinuation, innuendo, half-truths, and plain lies against an opponent; and in maintaining an efficient espionage system which could obtain reliable knowledge of the enemy's plans. Sometimes the required pressure could be applied through a man's business or professional connections; again, something might be accomplished through his family and relatives, in which case the local clergyman and the ladies of the W.C.T.U. were very helpful. (Asbury, 1968, pp. 101–102)

Not surprisingly one league leader would later write that the lies he told in promoting prohibition "would fill a big book" (Asbury, 1968, p. 102).

Decades later, their propaganda, strong organization, and political tactics would pay off in the passage of the Eighteenth Amendment to the U. S. Constitution establishing national prohibition. A leader of the Anti-Saloon League testified that prior to its passage in Congress, he had compiled a list of 13,000 business people who supported prohibition. They were then given their instructions at the crucial time:

We blocked the telegraph wires in Congress for three days. One of our friends sent seventy-five telegrams, each signed differently with the name of one his subordinates. The campaign was successful. Congress surrendered. The first to bear the white flag was Senator Warren Harding of Ohio. He told us frankly he was opposed to the amendment, but since it was apparent from the telegrams that the business world was demanding it he would submerge his own opinion and vote for submission. (Pollard, 1932, p. 107)

The league was so powerful that even national politicians feared its strength. The Eighteenth Amendment might well not have passed if a secret ballot had made it impossible for the league to have punished the "disobedient" at the next election (Sinclair, 1962, p. 110).

What was written about Wayne Wheeler, Counsel for the Anti-Saloon League was true, to a lesser degree, of many other temperance leaders:

Wayne B. Wheeler controlled six congresses, dictated to two presidents of the United States, directed legislation in most of the States of the Union, picked the candidates for the more important elective and federal offices, held the balance of power in both Republican and Democratic parties, distributed more patronage than any dozen other men, supervised a federal bureau from outside without official authority, and was recognized by friend and foe alike as the most masterful and powerful single individual in the United States. (Childs, 1947, p. 217)

The Civil War had interrupted the temperance movement while Americans were preoccupied with that great struggle. Then, after the war, the Women's Christian Temperance Union was founded. Of course, the organization did not promote moderation or temperance but rather prohibition. One of its methods to achieve that goal was education. It was believed that if it could "get to the children" it could create a dry sentiment leading to prohibition (Sheehan, 1981, p. 118).

ESTABLISHMENT OF ALCOHOL EDUCATION

Calls for alcohol education in the United States were heard as early as 1869, when a temperance writer, Julia Coleman, addressed the Fulton County (NY) Teachers' Institute on the subject (Mezvinsky, 1961, p. 48). Similar appeals were made by others over the next few years. In 1873 the National Temperance Society called for instruction in both public and private schools on the effects of alcohol on the human system (Mezvinsky, 1961, p. 48).

At about the same time, Mary Hunt, a former school teacher visited her local school board in Massachusetts and persuaded that body to establish temperance instruction in the schools. Then, together with Julia Coleman, Mrs. Hunt extended the campaign to other school districts in the state. They promoted a series of graded lessons on hygiene and physiology prepared by the former teacher (Ohles, 1978, p. 477) and a new textbook, *Alcohol and Hygiene*, authored by Ms. Coleman (Bordin, 1981, p. 135).

In 1879 Mrs. Hunt accepted an invitation from Frances Willard to speak to the WCTU's national convention on "Scientific Temperance Instruction." There she presented her vision of "thorough text-book study of Scientific Temperance in public schools as a preventive against intemperance" (Billings, 1903, p. 21). A standing committee was appointed with Mrs. Hunt as chair. The following year (1880) a Department of Scientific Temperance Instruction in Schools and Colleges, with Mrs. Hunt as National Superintendent, replaced the committee (Billings, 1903, p. 22).

In her new position, Mrs. Hunt called on each WCTU local to visit its school board to demand that temperance textbooks be incorporated into the regular course of study. Around the country, locals held mass meetings and petition drives converged on school boards to press their case. This led Mrs. Hunt to observe that "It is not too much to say that the school boards of the country . . . are in a state of siege" at the hands of WCTU members (Zimmerman, 1992, p. 2). She, herself, spoke to 182 meetings in 1880 (Ohles, 1978, p. 477).

But the results were disappointing to the WCTU. School boards were not as pliant as expected and it was much more difficult to remove recalcitrant board members. While Mrs. Hunt was having difficulty promoting her temperance instruction, the prohibition movement was experiencing serious difficulties as well. During the decade, 12 of 20 prohibition referenda were defeated and states were often failing to enforce those bills that did manage to pass. This led Mrs. Hunt to conclude that voters "must first be convinced that alcohol and kindred narcotics are by nature outlaws, before they will outlaw them" (Zimmerman, 1992, pp. 5–6). She decided to use legislation to coerce the moral suasion of students, who would be the next generation of voters. This gave birth to the idea of the compulsory Scientific Temperance Instruction Movement (Zimmerman, 1992, p. 6).

Mrs. Hunt's strategy was for WCTU members to pressure state legislators and promote the nomination and candidacy of pro-temperance candidates in election years. The strategy was first used in Vermont where highly organized members campaigned for temperance candidates, developed letter writing campaigns, obtained temperance endorsements from leading citizens, presented legislators with a deluge of petitions, and packed open hearings on a proposed bill. The strategy worked. The bill was passed by a large majority and became law in 1882 (Mezvinsky, 1961, p. 49). Mrs. Hunt developed and pioneered the use of tactics used ever since by lobbyists and pressure groups.

But Mrs. Hunt was not entirely pleased with her first effort; the Vermont law was general and vague. She feared that a few lessons presented to a few students could be interpreted as compliance with the law. Therefore, in the next state campaign, Mrs. Hunt worked to ensure that the proposed bill would require that temperance instruction be given to *all* students in *all* schools in Michigan (Mezvinsky, 1961, p. 49). One provision required schools to teach the harmful physical effects of alcohol, narcotics, and stimulants, while another required teachers to pass an examination on the effects of alcohol and narcotics. The Michigan law, passed in 1883, became a model for subsequent legislation in other states (Bordin, 1981, pp. 135–136).

Mrs. Hunt proved to be a brilliant strategist and leader. State prohibition laws had not been faring well and temperance could be a political minefield capable of destroying all but the most astute political operative:

Prohibition of alcohol was an issue that shook state politics in the nineteenth century. Even politicians in favor of temperance were not sure that they wanted to alienate voters by proscribing drink. Children, however, were another matter; they did not vote, and they might safely be taught to shun what their parents cared little to abandon. By the turn of the century every state and territory had laws mandating the teaching of the evils of alcohol.[6] Many of these laws were more specific and binding than legislation on any other branch of the curriculum. (Tyack and James, 1985, pp. 515–516)

However, many of the compulsory laws were still not strong enough to suit Mrs. Hunt. Even while some states were being pressured to enact legislation, she was waging campaigns to strengthen many of the existing laws. For example, due to Mrs. Hunt's continued efforts, Vermont's easily evaded 1882 legislation was amended in 1886. Even the model Michigan act was amended to include the same provisions as the revised Vermont law (Mezvinsky, 1961, p. 51). From there, Mrs. Hunt carried the amendment fight on to other states.

Not surprisingly, many school officials were unsympathetic or resistant to mandatory temperance education. An Ohio temperance worker complained that "school examiners, school boards and school superintendents are, many of them, indifferent to the law—ignore it—and are not dismissed" and observed that "no law will enforce itself" (Zimmerman, 1992, p. 8).[7] Accordingly, Mrs. Hunt asserted that "It is our duty not to take the word of some school official, but to visit the school and carefully and wisely ascertain for ourselves if the study is faithfully pursued by all pupils" (Zimmerman, 1992, p. 9). To this end, she asserted that local WCTU superintendents or other members must visit their local schools to observe the temperance lessons, examinations, recitations, and textbooks (Hunt, 1892, pp. 53, 58).[8] With about 150,000 members scattered in communities across the nation in 1892, the WCTU was in an excellent position to monitor compliance to the temperance legislation. "When, in an unusual gesture of defiance, teachers in New York State protested a highly prescriptive temperance law, the WCTU mobilized influential local members to make sure that teachers were obeying the statute" (Tyack and James, 1985, p. 517). Not surprisingly, both supporters and opponents used military metaphors to describe Hunt's organization and methods.

By the turn of the century, the Scientific Temperance Instruction movement directed by Mrs. Hunt had proved to be highly successful. Virtually every state, the District of Columbia, and all United States possessions had strong legislation mandating that all students receive anti-alcohol education. Some textbook authors even prepared different editions of their books to meet the differing legal requirements of various states (Nietz, 1961, p. 294). Furthermore, the implementation of this legislation was closely monitored down to the classroom level by legions of determined and vigilant WCTU members throughout the nation.

TEMPERANCE TEACHINGS

Enacting mandatory temperance instruction laws and making sure that they were strictly enforced was only part of the movement. Mrs. Hunt wanted to dictate the content of the instruction and textbooks. She was particularly disturbed that some of the texts being used were "not safe in that they did not preach total abstinence" and most did not devote at least one-fourth of their content to temperance instruction (Tyack and James, 1985, p. 517). She described her long search for acceptable texts as an "almost superhuman effort to secure absolute scientific accuracy, not modified in favor of occasional or moderate use of alcohol" (Bader, 1986, p. 99). But she was highly effective:

In 1886, after persuading Congress to require the use of a WCTU-approved text in Washington, D.C., and the territories, Hunt wrote a petition to publishers with a checklist for selecting textbooks that would comply with the temperance instruction laws. Books should stress, she said, that a little drink creates an uncontrollable craving for more, illustrate the "appalling effects of drinking habits upon the citizenship of the nation," and omit reference to the fact that doctors used alcohol for medicinal purposes. Temperance should not be relegated to an appendix; it should "be the chief and not the subordinate topic" in physiology texts, she wrote. WCTU members, following Hunt's lead, barraged publishers with petitions signed by school board officials and educators. Aware of the market being created by the new laws and eager to avoid offending the temperance lobby, seven major publishers promptly submitted their physiology texts to Hunt for review, while many others later decided it was best to have her endorsement. In 1891 she presented the WCTU convention with a list of twenty-five approved books. (Tyack and James, 1985, pp. 517–518)

The content of WCTU-approved textbooks can best be understood within the larger context of post-Civil War America with its rapid growth of science and quickly evolving temperance movement. In the decades following that war, increasing veneration for science occurred and medical research on the effects of alcohol flourished. In that environment:

the temperance societies set out to diffuse the results of medical research through pamphlet and pulpit. But they were careful to diffuse only that scientific data which was in line with their beliefs. The research which supported God's ban against drink was good; the research which found for the moderate use of liquor was faulty, biased, bought, or downright evil. The drys perfected techniques for misrepresenting scientific experiments, for quoting out of context, for making final dogmas out of interim reports, and for manufacturing literary water bottles out of laboratory test tubes. (Sinclair, 1962, pp. 38–39)

The scientific ideas promoted by temperance writers were clearly open to question. For example, before the Civil War they had enthusiastically taught the idea of spontaneous combustion of habitual drunkards. According to a temperance writer, "these cases of the death of drunkards by internal fires, kindled often spontaneously in the fumes of alcohol, that escape through the pores of the skin—have become so numerous and so incontrovertible, that I presume no person of information will now be found to call the reality of their existence into question (Krout, 1925, p. 232, superfluous commas in original). With the headline "Fire! Fire! Blood on Fire!," the *Pennsylvania Temperance Recorder* (February 1836) reported that a physician in Maine had touched a match to blood from a "common drunkard" and observed it burn for thirty seconds with a blue flame (Krout, 1925, p. 232). A schoolbook for children told the story of a man who was so full of alcohol that he exploded while attempting to light his pipe (Smith, 1844, p. 82). In spite of scientific refutation the idea had not died out as late as 1879 (E.M.J., 1941, p. 805), when a temperance writer described what he saw during a *post mortem* of a drunkard performed by two physicians: "After removing the top of the skull, for the purpose of examining the condition of the brain, they tested it for alcohol, by holding a lighted match near it; and immediately the brain took fire, and burned with a blue flame, like an alcohol lamp" (Asbury, 1968, p. 44, superfluous commas in original). Presumably the deceased's blood alcohol content far exceeded .10 percent!

A temperance leader explained the effects of alcohol on the body:

Dyspepsia, jaundice, emaciation, corpulence, dropsy, ulcers, rheumatism, gout, tremors, palpitation, hysteria, epilepsy, palsy, lethargy, apoplexy, melancholy, madness, delirium-tremens, and premature old age, compose but a small part of the catalogue of diseases produced by ardent spirit. Indeed, there is scarcely a morbid affection to which the human body is liable, that has not, in some way or another, been produced by it; there is not a disease but it has aggravated, nor a predisposition to disease which it has not called into action; and although its effects are in some degree modified by age and temperament, by habit and occupation, by climate and season of the year, and even by the intoxicating agent itself; yet, the general and ultimate consequences are the same. (Sewall, 1841, pp. 11–12)

The fate of the habitually intoxicated was inevitable and "everywhere the same. Its succession of horrible excesses constituted a form of suicide, the more terrible because death was preceded by excruciating mental and physical torture. Fortunate was the victim who sank into an untimely grave before he had been bereft of reason, or deprived of his physical powers" (Krout, 1925, p. 229).

Temperance advocates promoted the false idea that alcohol is not found in living organisms but only in decaying vegetable matter undergoing fermentation. They described it as resulting from death and decay, and asked: "Shall we turn away with loathing and disgust from the . . . vulture gorging itself with carrion all quivering with putrescence and then drink [wine] sparkling . . . by reason of a like work of decomposition going on within?" (Furnas, 1965, p. 195).

Temperance writers also skillfully manipulated language to manipulate thought and emotion. For example, alcohol is formed from the consumption of sugar by yeast and the by-product of this process can technically be described as an excrement, just as our breath carries the by-product or excrement of carbon dioxide created by our bodies and is technically also excrement. But since we ordinarily think of excrement as feces or urine, the temperance writers intentionally created disgust and loathing by describing alcohol as "the excretion of a fungus." Even the word fungus rather than yeast was chosen because of unpleasant association. So temperance writers and speakers could assert gleefully that fungi in grape juice "gorge themselves and leave their liquid excrement. That is what alcohol is. Now sing of your ruby wine!" (Furnas, 1965, p. 196).

Sometimes temperance advocates seem to have simply created facts out of thin air to make alcohol appear less desirable. One wrote that the famous nutty flavor of madeira was caused by dissolving a bag of roaches in the beverage (Krout, 1925, p. 164). The much less colorful reality is that the flavor is caused by oxidation of the wine (Baldy, 1993, p. 396).

As summarized in *The New American Cyclopaedia* of 1857:

The demand for prohibition, according to its advocates, logically rests on the assumption that alcohol is essentially a poison—precisely as arsenic, opium, and nicotine are poisons—that the difference between wine and brandy, beer and gin, a liquor containing five percent, and one containing fifty percent of alcohol, a glass of ale and a pint of rum, is one of degree merely, not of kind, at least so far as poison is concerned. They also argue in support of their position, that alcohol is a product of vegetable decay and dissolution, and hence necessarily hurtful—that there can be no temperate use of it as a beverage any more than there can be temperate theft, adultery, or murder—that, if much strong drink does great harm, a little weak alcohol drink must do some harm, and that there can be no temperate use of such beverages but their total disuse. (Ripley and Dana, 1857, p. 48)

Temperance materials made no distinction between drinking and alcohol abuse, which were portrayed as one and the same. A typical poster presented the virtue and blessings of the abstainer on one side and the sin and misery of the drinker (synonymous with the drunk) on the other. An important organ for the dissemination of temperance educational thought and practice was the *Temperance Educational Quarterly*:

In the Temperance Educational Quarterly, the advocates of prohibition described how temperance was to be taught in the public schools. Some articles gave scripts for teachers and pupils to use on Frances E. Willard day. Others printed pledges for children to sing in meetings modeled on revivalist principles. Others again told horror stories about drunkards and offered quotations from writers on the evils of liquor. The magazine featured prize essays by pupils on alcohol, smoking, and other evils and furnished detailed lesson plans. This pedagogy, like the textbooks approved by the WCTU, was one of moral absolutism, a luring world of virtue and vice. . . . Children were given "Thirty Scientific Facts" like these to recite:

Alcohol ruins the character.
Alcohol prevents men from obtaining good positions.
Nearly all business houses refuse to employ drinkers because they can not be trusted. They are careless, dull and irresponsible. (Tyack and James, 1985, p. 518)[9]

The textbooks endorsed by the WCTU reflected the view that "any quantity of alcohol in any form was toxic and when consumed regularly produced inheritable disorders into the third generation" (Kobler, 1973, p. 140). One such textbook asserted as "scientific" the idea that:

sometimes one is sick or suffers very much because of wrong things that his parents or grand-parents did. . . . Over in the poor-house is a man who does not know as much as most children four years old . . . because he is the child of drinking parents whose poisoned life blood tainted his own. Many men and women are insane because they inherit disordered bodies and minds, caused by the drinking habits of their parents; and the descendants of "moderate drinkers" differ in this way as well as those of the drunkard. . . . This is called the law of heredity . . . one of God's laws, and just like earthly laws, helps right living and punishes those who disobey. (Furnas, 1965, pp. 193–194)

Another approved textbook asserted that "One of the most destructive agents man has brought into use is alcohol" and explained:

It has often been observed that children of intemperate parents frequently fail to develop into manhood or womanhood. They may not be deformed, but their growth is arrested, and they remain small in body and infantile in character. . . . Such are examples of a species of degeneracy, and are evidences of the visiting of the sins of the fathers upon the children, which may extend even into the third and fourth generations. (Sheehan, 1984a, p. 104)

A temperance pamphlet, summing up allegedly accepted findings, stated that "the offspring of parents both of whom drink are invariably either insane, tuberculous or alcoholic" and cited cases of "small children with an hereditary yen for alcohol so strong that the mere sight of a bottle shaped like a whiskey flask brought them whining for a nip" (Furnas, 1965, p. 194).

Some temperance writers even implied that merely inhaling alcohol vapors might lead to defective offspring through their descendants for at least three generations (Ploetz, 1915, p. 29) and others expressed great concern for "racial welfare" (Ploetz, 1915, pp. 14–15; Gruber, 1910; Stehler, 191–) and called for "a hygiene of the life germs, race hygiene, eugenics, and [the] art of breeding (Gruber, 1910, p. 9).[10] Some of these and similar views would later be promoted by Adolf Hitler and Benito Mussolini (Morgan, 1988).

Suggested classroom demonstrations included putting part of a calf's brain in an empty jar into which alcohol would then be poured. The color of the brain would turn from pink to gray, and pupils would then be warned that a drink of alcohol would do the same to their brains (Kobler, 1973, p. 140). Or an egg could be cracked into a jar of pure alcohol and the curdled mess would be described as similar to the effect of alcohol on the stomach's lining (Sinclair, 1962, p. 39).

The WCTU's Department of Scientific Temperance Instruction promoted as scientifically proved fact that:

The majority of beer drinkers die from dropsy.
When it (alcohol) passes down the throat it burns off the skin leaving it bare and burning. It causes the heart to beat many unnecessary times and after the first dose the heart is in danger of giving out so that it needs something to keep it up and, therefore, the person to whom the heart belongs has to take drink after drink to keep his heart going.
It turns the blood to water.
[Referring to invalids], a man who never drinks liquor will get well, where a drinking man would surely die. (Kobler, 1973, p. 143)

The WCTU promoted compulsory temperance education so as to create "trained haters of alcohol to pour a whole Niagara of ballots upon the saloon" (Sinclair, 1962, pp. 43–44). To this end it required that textbooks which it approved "teach that alcohol is a dangerous and seductive poison; that fermentation turns beer and wine and cider from a food into poison; that a little liquor creates by its nature the appetite for more; and that degradation and crime result from alcohol" (Sinclair, 1962, p. 44).

At least one-fourth of each book had to consist of temperance teaching and publishers had difficulty selling textbooks that were not approved by the WCTU. "The cornerstone of the educational campaign was the absolute insistence that alcohol in any form and in any amount was a poison to the human system (Bader, 1986, p. 99). Many of the statements in approved texts were, at best, misleading and designed to frighten young impressionable readers:

The nature of alcohol is that of a poison . . . .
Any substance capable, when absorbed into the blood, of injuring health or destroying life, is a POISON. . . . Remember this—ALCOHOL IS A POISON. . . .
A cat or dog may be killed by causing it to drink a small quantity of alcohol. A boy once drank whiskey from a flask he had found, and died within a few hours. . . .
Any drink that contains alcohol is not a food to make one strong; but is a poison to hurt, and at last to kill . . . .
Alcohol is a colorless liquid poison. Its presence makes what was before a good fruit juice a poisonous liquid. (Alcohol) changes a food to a poison . . . alcohol and all spirituous liquors are poisonous. (Billings, 1903, pp. 30–31)

Not only did the approved textbooks describe alcohol as a poison; it was the cause of numerous physical problems and resulting death:

Very often in chronic, though perhaps moderate, drinkers, the arteries, instead of being strong, elastic tubes, like new rubber hoses, become hardened and unyielding, and are liable to give way.

[Among drinkers] in some cases the liver reaches an enormous weight, fifteen, and even twenty to twenty-five, pounds being not uncommon (Sheehan, 1984a, p. 105). Alcohol sometimes causes the coats of the blood vessels to grow thin. They are then liable at any time to cause death by bursting. . . . Worse than all, when alcohol is constantly used, it may slowly change the muscles of the heart into fat. Such a heart cannot be so strong as if it were all muscle. It is sometimes so soft that a finger could easily be pushed through its walls. You can think what would happen if it is made to work a little harder than usual. It is liable to stretch and stop beating and this would cause sudden death.

There is one form of . . . disease, called alcoholic consumption, which is caused by alcohol. The drinker looks well, till suddenly comes a "dropped stitch," or a pain in the side. Then follows difficulty of breathing and vomiting of blood, then a rapid passage to the grave. (Billings, 1903, pp. 32–33)

And the textbooks approved by the WCTU also implicated psychological problems as well:

Many people are made crazy by the use of alcoholic liquors. In some asylums where these people are kept, it has been found that nearly one half of the crazy people were made crazy from this cause. Not all of these were drinkers themselves. It often happens that the children of those who drink have weak minds or become crazy as they grow older . . . .

A noted murderer confessed that never, but once, did he feel any remorse. Then he was about to kill a babe, and the little creature looked up into his face and smiled. "But," he said, "I drank a large glass of brandy, and then I didn't care." (Billings, 1903, pp. 32–33)

The approved textbooks appear to have been written with the purpose of frightening children into avoiding all contact with alcohol. One can only speculate as to how many children unnecessarily suffered anxiety and emotional trauma as they watched their parents enjoy a glass of wine or a beer with their dinner. But the WCTU was unalterably opposed to moderation. Kobler (1973, p. 140) pointed out that:

Nowhere in all this gallimaufry of misguidance . . . aimed at children, or in any of the prohibition literature and talk addressed to adults, did there linger the ghost of a suggestion that perhaps one might drink moderately without damage to oneself or to others. The very word "moderation" inflamed the WCTU and the Prohibition Party. It was "the shoddy life-belt, which promotes safety, but only tempts into danger, and fails in the hour of need . . . the fruitful fountain from which the flood of intemperance is fed. . . . Most men become drunkards by trying to drink moderately and failing." Even conceding that a rare few could conceivably imbibe in moderation at no risk to themselves, they should nevertheless refrain lest they set a bad example for the weaker majority of the human race.

Thus, approved textbooks asserted that "To attempt to drink fermented liquors moderately has led to the hopeless ruin of untold thousands" and "It is the nature of alcohol to make drunkards" (Billings, 1903, pp. 30–31).

SCIENTIFIC TEMPERANCE INSTRUCTION CRITICIZED

By the mid-1890s, the extensive exaggerations, distortions, and gross inaccuracies in textbooks endorsed by the WCTU were increasingly criticized by leading scientists and educators. The latter included the presidents of Columbia, Cornell, Yale, Stanford, and Vassar (Mezvinsky, 1961, p. 52). Such criticisms became increasingly strong after a report issued by the prestigious Committee of Fifty, a group of leading citizens formed in 1893 by eminent sociologists to study the "liquor problem" (Furnas, 1965, p. 330). It sought to determine facts rather than promote any theory or point of view (Billings, 1905, p. 4). A subcommittee, headed by faculty from Harvard and Clark University, found the WCTU's program of temperance instruction seriously defective. The committee contended that children should not be taught and forced to memorize "facts" that they would later find to be incorrect. This instructional approach was seen as inappropriate and doomed to backfire.

By making such unqualified assertions as "Alcohol is a colorless liquid poison," the WCTU-approved textbooks clearly conveyed the false impression that alcohol is poison in any amount and is always harmful (Timberlake, 1963, p. 49). By constant repetition of the word poison and by making numerous exaggerations and false statements, the approved texts attempted to mislead and frighten young people into abstinence.[11]

The committee believed that instruction should be based on facts so that students could form their own educated opinions. They "should not be taught that the drinking of a glass or two of wine by a grown-up person is very dangerous" (Billings, 1905, pp. 35–36). This was diametrically opposed to the view expressed by a prominent WCTU leader that "To teach the danger of forming the awful, insidious, inexorable appetite [for alcohol], is the especial province of the teacher" (Bader, 1986, p. 100) and of Mrs. Hunt, who referred to the enormous "harvest of death that might result from the universal teaching that the drinking of one or two glasses of wine is not 'very dangerous'" and asserted that "such teaching would be nothing less than crime" (Hunt, 1904, pp. 17–18).

The committee contrasted contemporary knowledge on alcohol with that taught in WCTU-approved textbooks by placing side by side passages from standard authoritative textbooks with those from "Indorsed and Approved" textbooks (Billings, 1903, pp. 11–13, ellipses in original):

STANDARD TEXTBOOKS	"INDORSED AND APPROVED" TEXTBOOKS
"It may perhaps, be said with safety that in small quantities it (alcohol) is beneficial, or at least not injurious, barring the danger of acquiring an alcohol habit, while in large quantities it is directly injurious to various tissues."	"Alcohol is universally ranked among poisons by physiologists, chemists, physicians, toxicologists, and all who have experimented, studied and written upon the subject, and who therefore, best understand it."

"In practice we find that in many persons a small quantity of alcohol improves digestion; and that a meal by its means can be digested which would be wasted."

"The question of the propriety of the daily use of alcohol by healthy men is at present a very serious one, involving so many moral and politico-moral issues that is cannot be fully discussed here. Suffice it to state as obvious inferences from our present knowledge of the physiological action of alcohol, that the habitual use of moderate amounts of alcohol does not directly and of necessity do harm; that to a certain extent it is capable of replacing ordinary food, so that if it be scanty, or even if it be coarse and not easily digested, alcohol, in some form or other, is of great advantage; that in all cases it should be taken well diluted, so as not to irritate the stomach; and that wine or malt liquors are certainly preferable to spirits. . . ."

"As Lieben also found that this substance (alcohol) exists in the urine of dogs, horses, and lions, and as A. Rajewski obtained it from healthy rabbits, it must be acknowledged that our present knowledge strongly indicates that alcohol is formed and exists in the normal organism."

"Alcohol is not a food or drink. Medical writers, without exception, class alcohol as a poison."

"This alcohol is a liquid poison, a little of it will harm any one who drinks it, and much of it would kill the drinker."

"It must be remembered that in whatever quantity, or wherever alcohol is found, its nature is the same. It is not only a poison, but a narcotic poison."

". . . alcohol is often fatal to life. Deaths of men, women, and children from poisonous doses of this drug are common."

". . . when used as a beverage, it injures the health in proportion to the amount taken."

"This alcohol is poisonous. It is its nature, even in small quantities, to harm any one who drinks it. It is capable of ruining the character—as well as the health; and if one takes enough it will kill him."

One author of an approved series of textbooks remarked to the committee that "I have studied physiology and I do not wish you to suppose that I have fallen so low as to *believe* all those things I have put into those books" (Billings, 1903, p. 34, emphasis in original). While the author may not have fallen so low as to believe what he wrote, he did fall low enough to put it into textbooks for impressionable young students. However, it appears that relatively few authors were willing to compromise themselves by writing or revising books to conform to Mrs. Hunt's strict ideological guidelines, because one-third of the approved textbooks were written anonymously (Billings, 1903, p. 26). Mrs. Hunt had to pay one author $6,000 to write two books, an amount of money that could have built or purchased a very large and commodious house at that time. Furthermore, at least one of the texts "authored" by another writer has been attributed to Mrs. Hunt (American Library Association, 1973, v. 261, p. 17). By her own admission (Hunt, 1897, p. 49), the publisher of nearly all of the early written texts that were ultimately approved had asked her either to revise them herself or to supervise the revisions to bring them into conformity with WCTU guidelines.[12]

The investigating committee conducted a survey of all members of the American Physiological Society as well as of 45 physiologists, hygienists, and specialists in allied sciences holding prominent positions abroad. The goal was to "obtain valuable expert opinions from practically the entire scientific world" regarding Scientific Temperance Instruction (Billings, 1903, p. 14). Although a number of the scholars opposed the consumption of alcohol, every respondent from the American Physiological Society except one "oppose[d] the so-called 'scientific temperance instruction' as it is now being promoted in the schools, the strong conviction of a number being that it is resulting in more evil than good" (Billings, 1903, p. 15). Of the foreign scientists, only one reported being in support of the approved textbooks. "Even [August] Forel, perhaps the most energetic and brilliant advocate of total abstinence in Europe, who goes so far as to maintain that alcohol *in all doses* is a poison, remarks, in speaking of educational methods: 'I think that in America somewhat unwise methods have been adopted'" (Billings, 1903, p. 17, emphasis in original).

The committee expressed concern over the ideological and propagandistic nature of WCTU-approved textbooks and of the "Scientific Temperance Instruction" movement:

As is generally the case when feeling and prejudice run high, the temptation has been irresistible to either manufacture evidence or stretch it over points that it does not cover; to call "scientific" everything that happens to agree with [its] particular prejudices, and to relegate to the limbo of human error all the evidence that appears for the other side. Another characteristic feature of this movement has been the flattery of authors who favor the views to be inculcated with such appellations as "greatest living authority," "foremost scientist," "the wise physician of today, who is abreast of the modern investigations concerning the drug," "author of great prominence," "most skilled in his profession," "eminent scholar," etc. (Billings, 1903, p. 23)

While the WCTU and other temperance writers tended to exaggerate the stature of those who agreed with them, they "frequently . . . abused anyone who disagreed with them; indeed, derogatory and vituperative language became a trademark of the temperance crusade" (Isaac, 1965, p. 226). Frequently, they went beyond mere words. The Committee of Fifty noted "the efforts of the 'scientific temperance' people to secure the dismissal of state employees suspected of not being sufficiently in sympathy with their own extreme views" (Billings, 1903, p. 25), and Mrs. Hunt "pushed the editor of a temperance newspaper to investigate those opposed to temperance physiology instruction" (Pauly, 1990, p. 387).

After extensively documenting "'scientific temperance' propaganda" (Billings, 1903, p. 25), the committee noted that "It is little wonder that educators and teachers oppose 'scientific' temperance" (p. 31) because "the text-books are written with a deliberate purpose to frighten the children, the younger the better, so thoroughly that they will avoid all contact with alcohol" (p. 32). Indeed, a "study of what children actually remembered from their [Scientific Temperance

Instruction] physiology classes reported one pupil's response: Alcohol 'will gradually eat away the flesh. If anyone drinks it, it will pickle the inside of the body'" (Tyack and James, 1985, pp. 518–519).

The committee attempted to use contemporary social scientific methods to study alcohol and to avoid the moralism of the prohibitionists. It concluded that occasional and regular moderate drinking did not cause health problems, that drinking did not inevitably lead to drunkenness, and that alcohol education should be based on a recognition that "Intoxication is not the wine's fault, but the man's" (Billings, 1905, pp. 30, 35, 41).

The committee was clearly displeased about "the manner in which scientific authorities are misquoted in order to appear to furnish support to 'scientific temperance instruction'" (Billings, 1903, p. 35). Then, after reviewing the results of three studies of Scientific Temperance Instruction practice and outcomes, the committee concluded that "under the name of 'Scientific Temperance Instruction' there has been grafted upon the public school system of nearly all our States an educational scheme relating to alcohol which is neither scientific, nor temperate, nor instructive" (Billings, 1903, p. 44).

Mrs. Hunt prepared a *Reply to the Physiological Subcommittee of the Committee of Fifty* in which she charged the authors of the report with being prejudiced against abstinence instruction, blasted them for gross misrepresentation of facts, argued that alcohol *is* a drug, and insisted that the WCTU-endorsed textbooks were completely accurate. She then had the *Reply* entered into the *Congressional Record* (Hunt, 1904) and distributed more than 100,000 copies (Mezvinsky, 1959, p. 184).

THE LEGACY

It is indisputable that "By the time of her death in 1906, Mary Hunt had shaken and changed the world of education" (Ohles, 1978, p. 478) with her campaign for coercive temperance education (or "institutionalized prohibitionist propaganda" [Clark, 1965, p. 35]). In 1901–1902, 22 million school children were exposed to anti-alcohol education (Hunt, 1904, p. 23). "The WCTU was perhaps the most influential lobby ever to shape what was taught in public schools. Though it was a voluntary association, it acquired quasi-public power as a censor of textbooks, a trainer of teachers, and arbiter of morality" (Tyack and James, 1985, p. 519).

Temperance writers viewed the WCTU's program of compulsory temperance education as a major factor leading to the Eighteenth Amendment (Cherrington, 1920, p. 175; Colvin, 1926, pp. 178–179). Other knowledgeable observers agreed. For example, the U. S. Commissioner of Education asserted in 1920 that:

In the creation of a sentiment which has resulted first in local option, then in state prohibition, and now in national prohibition, the schools of the country have played a very important part, in fact probably a major part. . . . The instruction in physiology and hygiene with special reference to the effects of alcohol . . . has resulted first in clearer thinking, and second in better and stronger sentiment in regard to the sale and use of alcoholic drinks. (Timberlake, 1963, p. 46)

A study of legislative control of curriculum in 1925 indicated that teaching about temperance "is our nearest approach to a national subject of instruction; it might be called our one minimum essential" (Tyack and James, 1985, p. 516; also see Flanders, 1925).

The WCTU held a virtual monopoly over the selection of textbooks until the 1940s, when it began to experience competition from the Yale Center of Alcohol Studies (Mezvinsky, 1961, pp. 48–56). Writing in 1961, Mezvinsky (p. 54) reported that "some alcoholic physiology and hygiene textbooks still stress total abstinence. . . . Some schools still stage [temperance] assemblies and meetings each year and hold WCTU essay and oratorical contests." So-called Scientific Temperance Instruction "laid the groundwork for the formal drug education programs that remain high on the agendas of today" (Erickson, 1988, p. 333), and some of the laws Mrs. Hunt had passed still remain (Garcia-McDonnell, 1993, p. 13).

It can also be argued that compulsory Scientific Temperance Instruction failed to achieve its major objective of bringing about complete abstinence. Annual consumption of alcohol beverages increased between 1880 and 1920. That is, it increased between the beginning of the movement and the beginning of national prohibition. Additionally, the difficulty of enforcing prohibition and its ultimate failure indicates that the instruction had not convinced enough young people to abstain (and to support prohibition) when they became adults (Mezvinsky, 1961, p. 54).[13]

THE NOBLE EXPERIMENT

Mary Hunt (1897, p. 63) had expressed concern over "the enormous increase of immigrant population flooding us from the old world, men and women who have brought to our shores and into our politics old world habits and ideas [favorable to alcohol]" and peppered her writing with references to this "undesirable immigration" and "these immigrant hordes." She is but one example. The largely anti-foreign, anti-Catholic, anti-German, and anti-Semitic nature of the temperance movement has been extensively documented (Kobler, 1973, pp. 168–169; Odegard, 1928, pp. 24–35; Sinclair, 1962, ch. 2 and pp. 119–126; Stivers, 1983, p. 358; Hofstadter, 1965, pp. 289–290). It appears to be no coincidence that legislation restricting immigration occurred during the height of the temperance movement's power.

The strong anti-foreign prejudice during World War I, the argument that the alcohol beverage industry diverted grain needed for the war effort, the lack of organization on the part of the wets, the effective organization of the drys, and political intimidation all combined with the effects of decades of temperance propaganda to make possible the passage of the Eighteenth Amendment establishing national prohibition (Kobler, 1973, ch. 9; Kerr, 1985, ch. 6).

For decades, alcohol had been blamed for almost all human misery and misfortune. Salvation Army General Evangeline Booth summarized this belief:

> Drink has drained more blood,
> Hung more crepe,
> Sold more houses,
> Plunged more people into bankruptcy,
> Armed more villains,
> Slain more children,
> Snapped more wedding rings,
> Defiled more innocence,
> Blinded more eyes,
> Twisted more limbs,
> Dethroned more reason,
> Wrecked more manhood,
> Dishonored more womanhood,
> Broken more hearts,
> Blasted more lives,
> Driven more to suicide, and
> Dug more graves than any other poisoned scourge that
> ever swept its death-dealing waves across the world.
> (Seldes, 1960, p. 106)

Not surprisingly, for decades prohibition had been touted as the almost magical solution to the nation's poverty, crime, violence, and other ills (Aaron and Musto, 1981, p. 157). On the eve of prohibition the invitation to a church celebration in New York said "Let the church bells ring and let there be great rejoicing, for an enemy has been overthrown and victory crowns the forces of righteousness" (Asbury, 1968, p. 154). Jubilant with victory, some in the WCTU announced that, having brought prohibition to the United States, it would now go forth to bring the blessing of enforced abstinence to the rest of the world (Asbury, 1968, p.143; McCarthy and Douglas, 1949, p. 31). The leading prohibitionist in Congress confidently asserted that "There is as much chance of repealing the Eighteenth Amendment as there is for a hummingbird to fly to the planet Mars with the Washington Monument tied to its tail (Merz, 1969, p. ix).

The famous evangelist Billy Sunday staged a mock funeral for John Barleycorn and then preached on the benefits of prohibition. "The rein of tears is over," he asserted. "The slums will soon be only a memory. We will turn our prisons into factories and our jails into storehouses and corncribs" (Asbury, 1968, pp. 144–145). Since alcohol was to be banned and since it was seen as the cause of most, if not all, crime (Odegard, 1928, pp. 58–60), some communities sold their jails. One sold its jail to a farmer who converted it into a combination pig and chicken house while another converted its jail into a tool house (Anti-Saloon League of America, 1920, p. 28).

Unfortunately, hoping or even fervently believing would not make prohibition anything other than a great illusion. The actual consequences ranged from unfortunate to disastrous and deadly. Widespread disregard for law was obvious.

Within a week after the Eighteenth Amendment was imposed, small portable stills were on sale throughout the country (Asbury, 1968, p. 157). California's grape growers increased their acreage about 700 percent during the first five years of the noble experiment and production increased dramatically to meet a booming demand (Feldman, 1928, pp. 278–281). Grape juice was commonly sold as "bricks or blocks of Rhine Wine," "blocks of port," and so on along with a warning: "After dissolving the brick in a gallon of water, do not place the liquid in a jug away in the cupboard for twenty days, because then it would turn into wine" (Aaron and Musto, 1981, p. 159). One grape block producer was not quite so coy when it advertised:

Now is the time to order your supply of VINE-GLO. It can be made in your home in sixty days—a fine, true-to-type guaranteed beverage ready for the Holiday Season.
    VINE-GLO . . . comes to you in nine varieties, Port, Virginia Dare, Muscatel, Angelica, Tokay, Sauterne, Riesling, Claret and Burgundy. It is entirely legal in your home—but it must not be transported. (Cashman, 1981, p. 213)

The mayor of New York City even sent instructions on winemaking to his constituents (Aaron and Musto, 1981, p. 159). There was also wort, or beer that had been halted in the manufacturing process before the yeast was added. The purchaser added yeast, let the wort ferment, and then filtered it. Since wort was sold before it contained alcohol, it was legal and openly sold throughout the entire country (Asbury, 1968, p. 235). Often, the entire family would be involved in the production of home brews for illegal sale, as suggested by the following:

> Mother's in the kitchen
> Washing out the jugs;
> Sister's in the pantry
> Bottling the suds;
> Father's in the cellar
> Mixing up the hops;
> Johnny's on the front porch
> Watching for the cops.
> (Mendelson and Mello, 1985, p. 86)

And:

> Mother makes brandy from cherries;
> Pop distills whisky and gin;
> Sister sells wine from the grapes on our vine—
> Good grief, how the money rolls in!
> (Sinclair, 1962, p. 209)

Organized smuggling of alcohol from Canada and elsewhere quickly developed. "Rum rows" existed off the coasts of large cities where ships lined up just beyond the three mile limit to off-load their cargoes onto speed boats. Murder and hijacking were common in this dangerous but lucrative business. One of the most well known operators was Bill McCoy, who enjoyed a reputation for smuggling high quality beverages—the original "real McCoy" (Lender and Martin, 1982, p. 144).

There was also the notorious and ever-present organized bootlegging. The country's scourge led to massive and widespread corruption of politicians and law enforcement agencies and helped finance powerful crime syndicates. In addition to the murders of law enforcement officers there was an ever more common cause of death and disability caused by bootleggers:

highly toxic wood alcohols found their way into much of the available bootleg liquor. When denatured industrial alcohol was not sufficiently diluted, or was consumed in large quantities, the result was paralysis, blindness and death. In 1927, almost twelve thousand deaths were attributed to alcohol poisonings, many of these among the urban poor who could not afford imported liquors. In 1930, U.S. public health officials estimated that fifteen thousand persons were afflicted with "jake foot," a debilitating paralysis of the hands and feet brought on by drinking denatured alcohol flavored with ginger root. (Mendelson and Mello, 1985, p. 87)

A contemporary writer described "jake foot" or "jake paralysis":

The victim of "jake paralysis" practically loses control of his fingers. . . . The feet of the paralyzed ones drop forward from the ankle so that the toes point downward. The victim has no control over the muscles that normally point the toes upward. When he tries to walk his dangling feet touch the pavement first at the toes, then his heels settle down jarringly. Toe first, heel next. That's how he moves. "Tap-click, tap-click, tap-click, tap-click," is how his footsteps sound. . . . The calves of his legs, after two or three weeks, begin to soften and hang down; the muscles between thumbs and index fingers shrivel away. (Shepherd, 1930)

Many stills used lead coils or lead soldering, which gave off acetate of lead, a dangerous poison. Some bootleggers used recipes that included iodine, creosote, or even embalming fluid (Asbury, 1968, pp. 272–273, 283). The resulting problems caused financial burdens to the nation, but bootleg, being untaxed, deprived the treasury of much needed revenue.

Alcohol for industrial purposes could be legally produced. However, it was relatively easy to divert to illegal beverages. Therefore, the Prohibition Bureau tried to make it undrinkable by requiring the addition of one of 26 denaturants. Some, such as soft soap, were harmless, but others such as iodine, sulfuric acid, and wood alcohol, were poisonous. At least one-tenth of all industrial alcohol was ultimately drunk (Sinclair, 1962, pp. 200–201).

The New York legislature called on Congress to prohibit the use of harmful denaturants. But the Anti-Saloon League, the WCTU and others defended the use of wood alcohol and other poisons. Said one temperance leader, "the government is under no obligation to furnish people with alcohol that is drinkable when the constitution forbids it. The person who drinks this industrial alcohol is a deliberate suicide" (Asbury, 1968, p. 279).

The widespread corruption of public officials became a national scandal. Several rather typical cases reported by the *New York Times* in a short period illustrate the problem:

Fort Lauderdale, Florida—The sheriff, the assistant chief of police, and seventeen others, including policemen and deputy sheriffs, were arrested on charges of conspiracy.
Morris County, New Jersey—The former county prosecutor was found guilty of accepting bribes from liquor-law violators.
Philadelphia—A city magistrate was sentenced to six years in prison for accepting $87,993 in liquor graft during his ten months in office.
Edgewater, New Jersey—The mayor, the chief of police, two local detectives, a United States customs inspector, a New York police sergeant, and eight others were found guilty of conspiracy. A rum-runner confessed that he had paid them $61,000 to help land liquor worth one million dollars.
South Jacksonville, Florida—Practically the entire city administration, including the mayor, the chief of police, the president of the city council, the city commissioner, and the fire chief, were indicted by a federal grand jury. (Asbury, 1968, p. 187)

It became very difficult to convict those who violated prohibition because public support for the law and its enforcement eroded dramatically. For example, of 7,000 arrests in New York between 1921 and 1923, only 27 resulted in convictions (Lender and Martin, 1982, p. 154). That is a conviction rate of only one for every 260 arrests.

In addition to being ineffective, prohibition was counterproductive[14] because it encouraged the heavy and rapid consumption of high-proof distilled spirits[15] in secretive, nonsocially regulated and controlled ways. "People did not take the trouble to go to a speakeasy, present the password, and pay high prices for very poor quality alcohol simply to have a beer. When people went to speakeasies, they went to get drunk." (Zinberg and Fraser, 1985, p. 468). Zinberg and Fraser (1985, p. 470) conclude: "Removing the alcohol from the norms of everyday society increased drinking problems. Without well-known prescriptions for use and commonly held sanctions against abuse, prohibition drinkers were left almost as defenseless as were the South American Indians in the face of Spanish rum and brandy." They (1985, p. 470) suggest that prohibition "may have curtailed the growth of the responsible drinking practices that had emerged during the 25 or so years preceding Prohibition."

Near the end of prohibition an observer wrote that "Since 1920 [the beginning of prohibition] the changed attitudes of women toward liquor has been one of the most influential factors in the encouragement of lawless drinking. Drinking in 1910 was a man's game. . . ." He explained that "Drinking today is a man-and-woman's game. . . . In all former times the man got drunk and came home to his disgusted and long-suffering wife. Today they sometimes get drunk together and try to slip into the house as quietly as possible, so as not to wake the children" (Asbury, 1968, p. 159).

Some drinking establishments were not as respectable as the illegal and unregulated speakeasies. They included the "clip joint":

The typical clip joint was staffed by a bartender, two or three waiters who doubled as strong-arm men, a tough floor manager, a singer and a piano player, a half-naked cigarette girl, and from two to ten hostesses, depending upon the size of the place. The sucker was usually brought to the clip joint by a taxi driver or sent there by a hotel clerk; he was assured that he would find girls galore and lost of good liquor "right off the boat."

When he arrived he was immediately importuned to buy drinks for one or more of the hostesses, who intimated that they would be available for more interesting activities "after we get through work." The girls usually drank "gin highballs," which were compounded of water and a little orange juice or ginger ale, and for which the sucker was charged from one to two dollars. The sucker himself, for his initial drink, was given a double slug of raw alcohol doctored to resemble whiskey. If he got helplessly drunk, he was simply robbed and dumped into the gutter a block or so away from the clip joint. If through some miracle he remained fairly sober and showed a disposition to quit spending, the usual procedure was for one of the hostesses to accuse him of insulting her. Thereupon the floor manager would indignantly tell him to leave and present him with a bill, an outrageous compilation which included a large cover charge, a dozen drinks he hadn't ordered, all those he had already paid for, a bottle or two of liquor, a half dozen packs of cigarettes at a dollar each, and extras. If he paid, he was permitted to depart, although he was lucky if a sympathetic hostess didn't pick his pocket before he reached the door. If he protested, he was kicked and slugged until he was groggy or unconscious, after which he was robbed and thrown out. (Asbury, 1968, pp. 198–199)

Speakeasys, clip joints, and similar drinking establishments tended to replace the good restaurants in which people had earlier been able to dine leisurely and enjoy beverage alcohol in a moderate and restrained manner. Instead, they now gulped down highly alcoholic beverages that were untaxed, unregulated, and almost always dangerous to life and health.

Even as the problems caused by prohibition mounted and the political winds began to shift, drys sometimes became even more adamant in their support. The teetotaller Henry Ford wrote: "For myself, if booze ever comes back to the United States, I am through with manufacturing. . . . I wouldn't be interested in putting automobiles into the hands of a generation soggy with drink" (Willebrandt, 1929, p. 34). The president of the WCTU defended the actions of prohibition agents who clubbed a suspected bootlegger unconscious and then shot his wife as she ran to aid him, commenting tersely, "Well, she was evading the law, wasn't she?" (Lender and Martin, 1982, pp. 160–161). In response to contests for a solution to the problem of noncompliance with prohibition:

One woman suggested that liquor law violators should be hung by the tongue beneath an airplane and carried over the United States. Another suggested that the government should distribute poison liquor through the bootleggers; she admitted that several hundred thousand Americans would die, but she thought that this cost was worth the proper enforcements of the dry law. Others wanted to deport all aliens, exclude wets from all churches, force bootleggers to go to church every Sunday, forbid drinkers to marry, torture or whip or brand or sterilize or tattoo drinkers, place offenders in bottle-shaped cages in public squares, make them swallow two ounces of castor oil, and even execute the consumers of alcohol and their posterity to the fourth generation. (Sinclair, 1962, p. 26; for other suggestions, see Tietsort, 1929, ch. 8)

Fortunately, cooler heads prevailed. Even John D. Rockefeller, Jr., a lifelong abstainer who had contributed $350,000[16] to the Anti-Saloon League, announced his support for repeal because of the widespread problems caused by prohibition (Prendergast, 1987, p. 44; Kyvig, 1979, p. 96). He explained his change of belief in a letter published in *The New York Times*:

When the Eighteenth Amendment was passed I earnestly hoped—with a host of advocates of temperance—that it would be generally supported by public opinion and thus the day be hastened when the value to society of men with minds and bodies free from the undermining effects of alcohol would be generally realized. That this has not been the result, but rather that drinking has generally increased; that the speakeasy has replaced the saloon, not only unit for unit, but probably two-fold if not three-fold; that a vast array of lawbreakers has been recruited and financed on a colossal scale; that many of our best citizens, piqued at what they regarded as an infringement of their private rights, have openly and unabashedly disregarded the Eighteenth Amendment; that as an inevitable result respect for all law has been greatly lessened; that crime has increased to an unprecedented degree—I have slowly and reluctantly come to believe. (Kyvig, 1979, p. 152; Roizen, 1991, pp. 245–246)

The popular vote for repeal of prohibition was 74 percent in favor and 26 percent in opposition (Childs, 1947, pp. 260–261). So by a resounding three to one vote, the American people rejected prohibition; only two states opposed repeal (Merz, 1969, p. x). A hummingbird had indeed flown to Mars with the Washington Monument tied to its tail.

Billy Sunday had proclaimed John Barleycorn's death at the beginning of prohibition in 1920. But thirteen years later:

> the cheerful spring came lightly on,
> And showers began to fall;
> John Barleycorn got up again,
> And sore surprised them all.
> (Furnas, 1965, p. 337)

Happy throngs sang "Happy Days are Here Again!" and President Roosevelt would soon look back to what he called "The damnable affliction of Prohibition" (Blocker, 1976, p. 242). But not all were happy. The Anti-Saloon League declared "War . . . NO PEACE PACT—NO ARMISTICE" and warned that temperance forces would soon be ready to launch the "offensive against the liquor traffic" (Lender and Martin, 1982, p. 135).

ANOTHER TRY FOR PROHIBITION

While the president and most of the country recognized prohibition as a national disaster, clearly many temperance activists did not. Prohibition had been a major legacy of World War I (Rubin, 1979, p. 236, Clark, 1976, pp. 122–129; Timberlake, 1963, pp. 173–176) and, with war in Europe, temperance leaders again hoped to take advantage of the national emergency that would occur if the United States were drawn into that conflagration. One asserted that "the full force of dry pressure would once again be brought to bear on Congress" if we entered the war in order "to get as much prohibition as . . . possible" (Childs, 1947, p. 219). Stressing that World War I had been the impetus for prohibition, a protemperance journal predicted promising times ahead (Rubin, 1979, p. 237).

After the United States was attacked, temperance leaders tried to have all alcohol prohibited on all military bases. One dry leader said, "I would rather have a sober son in a concentration camp in Germany than in a service camp in America if that son should become the victim of the drink habit" (Rostow, 1942, pp. 230–231). However, the Secretary of War insisted that "temperance cannot be attained by prohibition," and supported the sale of beer and light wine on military bases. He believed that this policy had "caused a degree of temperance among Army personnel which is not approachable in civil communities now" by encouraging soldiers "to remain on the reservation (their home) and enjoy refreshment under conditions conducive of temperance" (Rubin, 1979, pp. 238–239). Similarly, Army Major Merrill Moore called for policies to encourage moderation among soldiers who chose to drink and asserted: "Not alcohol, but the intemperate use of alcohol, is the problem in the Army as well as in civilian life" (Moore, 1942, p. 249). The Office of War Information pointed out that bootleggers could not be regulated whereas legal dispensers could (Rubin, 1979, p. 253).

Furthermore, the availability of beverage alcohol was seen by military authorities as good for morale and the war effort. Brewers were required to allocate 15 percent of total annual production of beer for use by the armed forces; local draft boards were authorized to grant deferments to brewery works who were highly skilled and irreplaceable; the Teamsters were ordered to end a strike against Minneapolis breweries because beer manufacturing was considered an industry essential to the war effort; and near the end of the war, the army made plans to operate recaptured French breweries to ensure adequate supplies for the troops (Rubin, 1979, p. 240).

An editorial in the daily newspaper of the U.S. Armed Forces in Europe, *The Stars and Stripes*, expressed alarm at temperance activities back home in the United States. It observed that:

Taking advantage of wartime conditions and restrictions, the new prohibition group is working night and day for legislation which will give America prohibition in fact if not in name. . . .

We can remember the days of prohibition, when moonshine whiskey made quick fortunes for bootleggers, crooked politicians and dishonest police officials. As a result we claim we know what we want in the way of liquor legislation and feel those at home should wait until we return before initiating further legislation on liquor control. (Childs, 1947, pp. 248–249)

Perhaps in the belief that the end justifies the means, temperance leaders frequently made clearly erroneous assertions. For example, a leading dry editor wrote that "The liquor interests use more than 1,250,000 tons of sugar every year, which is more than the one-half pound ration per week for every man, woman and child in the United States of America" (Childs, 1947, p. 224). Actually, no sugar is used in producing distilled spirits beverages. Similarly, the president of the

WCTU wrote that "Total consumption of legal and illicit liquor in the fiscal year ended June 30, 1941, was approximately 2, 017,835,015 gallons," (Childs, 1947, p. 225). That would have been over 15 gallons for every man, woman, and child in a country that contained a large proportion of abstainers!

Dry leaders insisted that Congress prohibit the production of alcohol beverages for at least the length of the war, arguing that intoxication caused the disaster at Pearl Harbor, wasted precious raw materials, reduced efficiency through excessive absenteeism, and would lead to loose lips among those with military secrets. But Congress would not be swayed this time (Rubin, 1979, pp. 245–246).[17]

TEMPERANCE MOVEMENT BIDES ITS TIME

Writing shortly after World War II, Childs (1947, p. 229) observed that, according to national opinion surveys, "About one-third of the people of the United States favor national prohibition." He explained (p. 229) that:

The prohibition forces are well organized and adequately financed. They carry on persistent propaganda against the sale and use of alcoholic beverages. Their long-range plan is, first, to dry up local communities by local option elections; second, when feasible, to bring about state prohibition; and, third, in the future, to restore national prohibition.

National prohibition had been repealed by the Twenty-first Amendment which contains two short but important sentences:

Section 1: The eighteenth article of amendment to the Constitution of the United States is hereby repealed.
Section 2: The transportation or importation into any State, Territory, or Possession of the United States for delivery or use therein of intoxicating liquors, in violation of the laws thereof, is hereby prohibited.

Section one made it again legal to import, produce, and sell beverage alcohol, while section two delegated to the States authority for regulating such beverages. The federal government did, however, retain the authority to tax alcohol and it soon asserted regulatory authority at the national level. The government now regulates alcohol largely through the Bureau of Alcohol, Tobacco, and Firearms of the Department of the Treasury. The bureau's functions include issuing basic permits to importers, warehouses, manufacturers, and wholesalers to conduct business; interdiction of illicit alcohol; and regulation of labeling and advertising of alcohol beverages (Mendelson and Mello, 1985, pp. 93–94).

Upon repeal of national prohibition, 18 states continued prohibition at the state level. The last state finally dropped it in 1966. Almost two-thirds of all states adopted some form of local option which enabled residents in political subdivisions to vote for or against local prohibition. Therefore, despite the repeal of prohibition at the national level, 38 percent of the nation's population lived in areas with state or local prohibition (Mendelson and Mello, 1985, p. 94).

Currently, about one-third of all states have adopted the control or state monopoly system, in which state government owns and operates all wholesale and retail alcohol beverage sales. The rest of the states use the license system, in which the state licenses and regulates all wholesalers and retailers.

It is obvious that:

The confusion and warped attitudes engendered by this long and bitter struggle [over prohibition] have not disappeared. National prohibition is dead, but the movement is still with us under different names. The fifty states have varied and even conflicting laws; for example, in one state food must be served in the same place as liquor, while in an adjoining state not one but two walls must separate food from liquor. A few counties in local-option states are legally dry. Attitudes toward law and authority still suffer as an aftermath. Drinking and drunkenness are still equated by some, with moralistic implications contrary to the concept of alcoholism as a disease. (Royce, 1981, p. 42)

During the Vietnam conflict, increased political pressure arose to lower the minimum drinking age. It was commonly argued that if soldiers were old enough to go to war and endanger their lives for their country, then they were old enough to purchase and consume a can of beer. This, combined with the increasing political activism of young people, led to the lowering of the drinking age in many states (Lotterhos et al., 1988, p. 632).

With the passage of time, heightened concern was expressed over problems related to the misuse of alcohol. Increased auto accidents and fatalities among young drivers were attributed to the lower legal drinking ages. While these increases may have resulted from greater use of cars or other factors, they were popularly blamed on the lower drinking ages. Highly publicized fears about the possible negative impact of alcohol on the health and well-being of citizens often exaggerate justifiable concerns and ascribe blame to alcohol without considering other contributing factors (Mendelson and Mello, 1985, p. 98). In politics, it is the perception of reality (rather than reality) that drives legislative action (Hanson, 1990, p. 89).

Americans are becoming more health and safety conscious. A preliminary report suggesting the mere possibility that oat bran might be helpful in reducing heart disease can create a dramatic increase in consumer demand for food products containing that product. The suggestion that a chemical sprayed on apple trees might be associated with cancer in rats if it is consumed in massive quantities can cause widespread fear and a dramatic reduction in demand for that fruit. Headlines incorrectly linking alcohol with a health or social problem can have a profound affect on behavior, and even on public policy.

THE NEW TEMPERANCE MOVEMENT

The existence of the National Institute of Alcoholism and Alcohol Abuse (NIAAA), the federal Center for Substance Abuse Prevention (CSAP),[18] and state alcohol abuse agencies has been beneficial in many ways. But it has also "engendered bureaucratic incentive for convincing the people and members of

Congress (who appropriate funds) of the perils and dangers of contemporary alcohol problems" (Mendelson and Mello, 1985, pp. 98–99). The welfare and survival of the alcohol agencies depends largely on promoting the widespread belief that alcohol problems are enormous, are growing, and are a serious burden on the economy.

While such agencies typically state as fact that alcohol is responsible for half of all traffic deaths in the United States, this statistic has no solid foundation. That figure typically includes all traffic fatalities that involve anyone (passengers, for example) who has consumed any alcohol. The most accurate estimates, however, from the unbiased National Academy of Sciences, are that roughly one-quarter of fatal accidents are caused by intoxication (Ross and Hughes, 1986). Similarly, estimates of the number of auto accidents that might involve alcohol in any way (passenger, pedestrian, etc.) become transformed into statistics on the number of accidents that are actually caused by drunk drivers (Zylman, 1974, p. 64). This, in spite of estimates that "about one half of the fatal road accidents involving a drunk driver would have occurred even if all drivers had a zero blood alcohol level" (Room, 1985, p. 12).

In addition to exaggerating the extent of drinking problems, alcohol agencies distort the costs of alcohol abuse by basing estimates on questionable assumptions, by confusing correlation with causality, by looking only at costs while ignoring the economic benefits of alcohol and by not using sound accounting principles (Wiener, 1981, pp. 185–188; Ford, 1988, pp. 134–165). However, the agencies' seriously flawed and inflated estimates are routinely presented to the American public as factual knowledge (Hein and Pittman, 1989).

Estimates by independent researchers of the number of people who have experienced any drinking problems within the previous three years as well as those of the number likely ever to experience a problem in the future have been transformed into agency assertions of the actual number of problem drinkers (Mulford, 1982, pp. 453–454) in spite of protests by the researchers concerned with the distortions and misuse of their data (Cahalan, 1979). The motives of the alcohol agencies are clear. It would appear that one is an attempt to justify the existence of jobs while the other is to expand bureaucratic budgets and power.

In 1980, Mothers Against Drunk Driving (MADD) was formed and the next year Students Against Driving Drunk (SADD) was established. Shortly thereafter, the National Transportation Safety Board recommended that states raise the legal drinking age to 21 (Blocker, 1989, pp. 164–165).

During the 1980s, advocacy groups such as the Center for Science in the Public Interest, the National Coalition for the Prevention of Impaired Driving and the National Council on Alcoholism and Drug Dependency pressed for legislation to limit and reduce the consumption of beverage alcohol (Engs, 1991, p. 156). By 1987, political pressure led to a federally mandated expansion (under threat of withholding highway funds) of alcohol prohibition in all states to all citizens under the age of 21. This was followed in 1991 by a federal tax increase on alcohol beverages, and state laws reducing the acceptable blood alcohol content for driving. Anti-alcohol policies have led to a dramatic decrease in beer, wine, and spirits consumption since 1980 (Hanson, 1995b). But lower is never low enough. As a neo-dry critic wrote, "The slogan for the new temperance is, regarding alcohol, 'less is better'" (Beauchamp, 1987, p. 62). Not surprisingly, "Attitudes toward alcohol in the 1990s are more intolerant than at any time since the early 1930s" (Rorabaugh, 1991, p. 19).

It is clear that:

In contemporary America, both the tactics and the tone of temperance sentiment have changed appreciably from the 1800s. Inebriety, licentiousness, moral depravity and sin have all but vanished form the extant vocabulary. The new contender for the status of moral purity would seem to be health (although ill-health has not yet achieved equivalence with religious fundamentalists' conceptions of sin). Today, rallying cries once structured in terms of social order, home and basic decency are now framed in terms of health promotion and disease prevention. (Mendelson and Mello, 1985, p. 99)

The temperance movement never really died. It was relatively dormant for several decades after World War II, but has re-emerged with a new identity and modified ideology. It has been described as "neo-prohibition" (Pittman, 1980), "new temperance" (Beauchamp, 1987; Heath, 1989; Blocker, 1989, p. 158), "new Sobriety" (Page, 1991), "new Victorianism" (Heath, 1989), and "new paternalism" (Gusfield, 1985, p. 76). The renewed movement is based on the assumption that individuals cannot be trusted to make appropriate lifestyle choices. Therefore, "to protect people from themselves or to protect society, the state should pass legislation that enforces restrictions likely [in the belief of the reformers] to promote health by taking away the individual's personal choice" (Engs, 1991, p. 156). This, in spite of the fact that alcohol legislation in the United States already appears to be among the most stringent in the world (Mosher, 1980).

SUMMARY

Alcohol has been part of American life since the beginning of the colonies. European settlers viewed alcohol as the "good gift of God," to be used and enjoyed in moderation by young and old alike; however, its abuse was neither approved nor tolerated and was seen as being "from the Devil." Both formal and informal controls enforced moderation, which was the typical pattern of consumption.

The Revolutionary War brought about dramatic social changes that reduced control over alcohol abuse. Drunkenness increased at the very time a changing and industrializing economy required a reliable work force. Simultaneously, many of the problems caused by industrialization, urbanization, and other changes were blamed on the new phenomenon of frequent intoxication.

As a result, a movement then arose to encourage the moderate or temperate use of alcohol. But with the passage of time, most temperance groups began to insist that no one should be permitted to drink any alcohol. Temperance came to mean prohibition and the good gift of God came to be seen as the evil Demon Rum.

After the Civil War, churches increasingly began to view prohibition as a religious issue and fought for it as a holy crusade against sin. Churches were joined in their crusade by numerous women's groups—alcohol was considered a defiler of women and destroyer of families and home life. The Women's Christian Temperance Union initiated a successful campaign to mandate legally the teaching of temperance (termed Scientific Temperance Instruction) throughout the entire public education system. After carefully examining the mandated curriculum, a prestigious body of scientists and educators concluded that Scientific Temperance Instruction was neither scientific, temperate, or instructive. In spite of these and many other objections, temperance instruction continued unabated and was later credited with contributing to the rise of national prohibition in 1920.

The noble experiment of national prohibition began with the optimistic belief of temperance workers that it would bring about a dramatic reduction in the nation's poverty, crime, and other social problems. Unfortunately, it was not to be. To the contrary, prohibition brought about a dramatic increase in organized crime, the extensive consumption of dangerous bootleg alcohol, widespread corruption of public officials, general disrespect for law, and an increase in the rapid consumption of high proof alcohol beverages. Recognizing the disastrous problems caused by prohibition, the American people called for its repeal by a resounding three to one margin.

But repeal did not eliminate support for prohibition. A substantial minority of the population maintained its strongly anti-alcohol sentiments and many tried to use World War II as an excuse to reimpose prohibition to whatever degree possible. While its goal was largely defeated, the temperance movement continued to exist and promote its cause. However, it was largely dormant for several decades.

By 1980, temperance sentiment re-emerged in a new guise. Variously referred to as the new temperance, the neo-dry, the neo-prohibition, and similar terms, this most recent incarnation has modified its ideology and political strategy. The next chapter describes in more detail this growing and very powerful new temperance movement.

NOTES

1. Except for several tribes in the Southwest, Native Americans did not have alcohol beverages before their introduction by Europeans in the 1600s. The Apache and Zuñi drank alcoholic beverages which they produced for secular consumption, while the Pima and Papago produced alcohol for religious ceremonial consumption. Although Papago consumption was heavy, it was limited to a single peaceable annual ceremony and the drinking among other groups was also infrequent and not associated with any drinking problems (MacAndrew and Edgerton, 1969).

2. First Timothy 4:4; Matthew 15:11; Luke 7:33–35.

3. Tavern owners typically enjoyed high status in the community, as indicated by the early records of Harvard. There, where names of students were listed according to the social position of their fathers, tavern owner's sons preceded those of the clergy (Krout, 1925, p. 44).

4. "Treasury Secretary Alexander Hamilton saw the whiskey makers as a good potential source of revenue to pay the enormous debt inherited by the Young Republic. In 1791, Congress enacted an excise tax on distilled spirits, a tax that fell heavily on the mountain

distillers of western Pennsylvania. The ensuing violence was known as the Pennsylvania Whiskey Rebellion" (Mendelson and Mello, 1985, p. 17).

5. One observer has noted that:
    There are many senses of the word *temperance*. It is traditionally used to translate *sophrosune*, Aristotle's virtue of moderation in the sphere of food, drink and sex; a virtue which, like all Aristotle's moral virtues, lies between a vice of excess and one of deficiency. Again, there is the familiar narrow Victorian sense of the word, which applies only to alcohol and signifies not moderation but complete abstinence; through the process which philosophers call persuasive definition, the favourable connotations belonging to an emotive word of rather vague meaning became attached to a new, specific content (Telfer, 1990, p. 157).

6. Mrs. Hunt asserted in 1904 (p. 3) that such education was "now mandatory in the public schools of every state in the United States, and in all schools under Federal control." However, Billings (1903, p. 100) reported that Georgia was "the only State having no law on the subject" while Flanders (1925, p. 68) reported that "Idaho was then [1903] the only state where it [temperance instruction] was not prescribed." But Billings (1903, p. 100) presented section eight of the relevant act, which had become Idaho law in 1899.

7. A pamphlet prepared by the superintendent of Kansas' Scientific Temperance Instruction Department and sent to every public school teacher in that state asserted that they *must* impress upon their students the important fact, which she asserted had been established by science indisputably beyond question, "that the use of alcoholic beverage *at all* is an abuse of the human system in exactly the proportion to the amount taken" (Bader, 1986, p. 100, emphasis in original).

8. Not surprisingly, it would appear that many teachers resented this intrusion into their professional autonomy. As one WCTU "compliance monitor" reported, "None of [them] have taken very kindly to the new departure of being watched, questioned or advised by their constituents" (Zimmerman, 1992, p. 20).

9. Sinclair (1962, p. 425) noted that:
    Even toddlers in Sunday schools were not exempt from warnings about the connection of alcohol and venereal diseases. Mrs. Wilbur F. Crafts, in her "Blackboard Temperance Lessons," suggested that a Temperance Knight be drawn on the blackboard, armored with various protections against the assaults of King Alcohol. When referring to the piece of armor which covered the knight's private parts, the teacher was to say, "King Alcohol has killed off a lot of people by wounding them in the part of the body that I have covered with the waist piece."

10. One can only speculate as to what may have passed for science at the American Temperance University, which existed for a time in the dry town of Harrisman, Tennessee (Furnas, 1965, p. 325).

11. The American Alcohol Education Association would later teach that alcohol is a "protoplasm poison" (Furnas, 1965, p. 317), a description that was apparently seen as sounding more scientific.

12. More specifically, the seven publishers agreed to amend their texts on the condition that Mrs. Hunt would revise them or supervise their revision. While she claimed that she never took money for a book endorsement, "she considered it only right that she be compensated for the labor necessary to bring an 'imperfect' book up to her particular scientific and pedagogical standards" (Pauly, 1990, p. 373). Significantly reflecting her character and lack of integrity was the fact that:

In order to deal with the accusation that she profited from reform, she signed over to charity the royalties due her on the thousands of physiology textbooks sold annually. Yet she believed that philanthropy began at home; her never-publicized beneficiary was the Scientific Temperance Association, a group composed of Hunt, her pastor, and a few friends. The association used its funds to support the operations of the national headquarters of the WCTU's Department of Scientific Temperance Instruction, a large house in Boston that was also Hunt's residence. (Pauly, 1990, p. 373)

13. With the institution of prohibition in 1920, the WCTU enlarged its Scientific Temperance Instruction campaign even more because of its fear that not enough people were convinced of the evil of alcohol (Ormond, 1929, p. 11).

14. Prohibition was similarly ineffective and counterproductive in Russia (1916–1917), Finland (1919–1932), Iceland (1919–1932) (Ewing and Rouse, 1976, p. 27), Belgium, England, Norway, Austria (Mendelson and Mello, 1985, p. 83), and elsewhere around the world (Heath, 1987, p. 46; Marshall, 1979, 456). Cross-culture evidence suggests that "The only 'prohibition' against alcohol consumption that seems to work in human society is that taken on *voluntarily* by the drinker himself" (Marshall, 1979, p. 456, emphasis in original).

15. Distilled spirits are more easily concealed and smuggled than are bulkier beer and wine. The resulting increased consumption of the more potent spirits has been called the iron law of prohibition (Cowan, 1986; see also Thornton, 1991, especially pp. 100–105).

16. Levine (1985) suggested that Rockefeller contributed over $700,000 to the Anti-Saloon League between 1900 and 1919 while Thornton (1991, p. 52) wrote that "unsubstantiated claims place that figure in the tens of millions of dollars." However, even the $350,000 figure represented an enormous sum of money during the early part of the century, when the typical head of a household earned $9 to $12 per week (Ziegler et al., 1911, p. 61).

17. The tactics of the new prohibition movement were described in detail at the time (Lee, 1944).

18. The Center for Substance Abuse Prevention is the newer name for the Office for Substance Abuse Prevention.

2

Issues
in
Alcohol Education

The prohibitionist impulse has reemerged in a new guise: control-of-consumption. This neo-dry movement currently calls for policies to discourage and reduce the consumption of alcohol, which it views as an undesirable substance. The contrasting sociocultural approach, based on the positive experience of Italians, Jews, Greeks, and many others around the world, argues that the problem is not alcohol but the misuse of alcohol. It calls for policies to reduce alcohol abuse. In addition to deciding whether to follow a control-of-consumption (more accurately, a reduction-of-consumption) or a sociocultural approach, educators developing alcohol education curricula are faced with decisions regarding the specific program objectives, the target group or groups, the teaching personnel to be used, and the content and methods to be employed.

PROHIBITION REDEFINED BY NEO-DRYS AS A GREAT SUCCESS

A recent magazine article on alcohol states that:

Prohibition Didn't Work

What everyone knows about prohibition is that it was a failure. It did not eliminate drinking. It did create a black market. That, in turn, spawned criminal syndicates and random violence. Corruption and widespread disrespect for the law were incubated and, most tellingly, Prohibition was repealed only 14 years after it was enshrined in the Constitution. But the conventional view is not supported by the facts. (Hammond, 1994, pp. 13–14)

Readers are treated to a rosy account of prohibition's success almost as glowing and far-fetched as the following:

Prohibition did not fail. On the contrary, it was a tremendous success. . . . It brought significant gains to society as a whole and made life more livable for many American families. . . . America prospered economically during the Prohibition period . . . it actually brought about a marked decrease in crime of all kinds (Methodist editor, 1970, p. 3).

Even the Federal Office for Substance Abuse Prevention (OSAP) (Resnik, 1990) has described prohibition as a success in protecting Americans from the "dangerous drug of alcohol," as have some neo-temperance writers (for example, Moore, 1989; Schwartz, 1990, p. 5; Prendergast, 1987, pp. 42–44; Gross, 1983, p. 8; Single, 1988, p. 337). They have apparently forgotten the many blessings of illegal bootleg with its resulting "jake paralysis," illness, blindness, and death.[1]

THE CONTROL-OF-CONSUMPTION APPROACH[2]

These views are consistent with the neo-dry or control-of-consumption approach to reducing alcohol problems. This orientation—sometimes called the control-of-production, the availability, the new temperance, the neo-prohibitionist, or the public health model—tends to assume that:

1. The substance of alcohol is in and of itself the complete and total cause of all drinking problems.
2. The availability of alcohol determines the extent to which it will be consumed.
3. The quantity of alcohol consumed (rather than the manner in which it is consumed, the purpose for which it is consumed, the social context in which it is consumed, etc.) determines the extent of drinking problems.
4. Educational efforts should be directed toward stressing the problems that alcohol consumption can cause and encouraging abstinence.

The more traditional control-of-consumption approach called for the complete and total prohibition of the manufacture, distribution, sale, possession, or consumption of any and all beverage alcohol. Given the clear failure of prohibition, supporters of the control-of-consumption model more typically call for a variety of measures designed to discourage consumption. These include much practices as:

- imposing higher taxes on alcohol beverages,
- limiting or reducing the number of sales outlets,
- restricting even more the permissible locations for sales outlets,
- limiting the alcohol content of beverages,
- prohibiting or restricting the advertising of alcohol,
- prohibiting or restricting the promotion of alcohol (through sponsorship of athletic events, sponsoring events on college campuses, giving free samples, etc.),
- requiring the use of warnings with all advertisements and commercials,
- requiring the use of stronger warning labels on all beverage containers,
- requiring the display of stronger warning signs in establishments that sell or serve alcohol beverages,
- limiting the days or hours during which alcohol can be sold,
- increasing server liability for subsequent problems associated with the misuse of alcohol,

- limiting the sale of alcohol to people of specific ages,
- decreasing the legal blood alcohol content level for driving vehicles or operating equipment, and
- eliminating the tax deductibility of alcohol as a business expense.

The control-of-consumption approach assumes that the problem is alcohol rather than the abuse of alcohol. Therefore, it attempts to discourage or prevent people from consuming alcohol rather than trying to prevent them from using alcohol irresponsibly. A leader in the alcohol field wrote that even after all these decades following the end of prohibition "we are being advised to enact inhibition," and suggested an explanation for the view that the problem is alcohol itself rather than the abuse of alcohol:

the alcoholismists—with still mainly alcoholics in their ranks and leadership—are in full cry against alcohol. I have heard the foremost leader among them say, "if it hadn't been for alcohol, I would never have become an alcoholic." What he meant was, alcohol is the cause of alcoholism. And that is what many alcoholics would like to believe: that, of course, there was nothing wrong with them; that they were not primarily weak or deficient; that alcohol just happened to get the best of them. Once they stopped the alcohol, they were all right. So alcohol was the cause. (Keller, 1985, p. 170)

Consistent with this restrictive approach was the action of one house of the Mississippi legislature in passing legislation to raise the minimum drinking age to 50 (Mosher, 1980, p. 31). Even more consistent would be raising it to the retirement age of 65 or the average life expectancy age of 74 (Famighetti, 1995, p. 972). A much more accurate term for the approach would be *reduction*-of-consumption.

ALCOHOL STIGMATIZED BY REDUCTION-OF-CONSUMPTION ADVOCATES

Under the direction of Ernest Noble, the National Institute on Alcohol Abuse and Alcoholism (NIAAA) adopted the reduction-of-consumption approach in the late 1970s. (National Institute on Alcohol Abuse and Alcoholism, 1978, p. 48). In Noble's opinion, "Alcohol is the dirtiest drug we have. It permeates and damages all tissue. No other drug can cause the same degree of harm that it does. Not even marijuana, heroin or LSD, as dirty and dangerous as they are, are as pervasive in the damage they cause as alcohol" (Ford, 1988, p. 176). The institute's deputy director has publicly asserted that there is no such thing as responsible drinking, and the Secretary of the Department of Health and Human Services has directed all agencies under his direction to replace the phrase "substance abuse" with "alcohol and other drug abuse" (Ford, 1988, p. 176). Federal officials seem to have taken their cue from Mary Hunt and other temperance zealots. As an alcohol educator observed decades ago, "The temperance publications to discourage drinking have associated alcohol with drugs in the hope that the social stigma and fear attached to drug addiction would also become identified with the use of alcohol. Legislation requiring schools to provide instruction about alcohol frequently incorporates the phrase 'alcohol and other narcotic drugs'" (McCarthy, 1959, p. 26). The federal Office for Substance Abuse Prevention's editorial guidelines (New York State Divisio of Alcoholism and Alcohol Abuse, n.d.a., p. 77) include the following:

Do Not Use	**Use**
Substance abuse	Alcohol and other drug abuse
Substance use	Alcohol and other drug use
Abuse when sentence refers to youth, teens, or children (anyone under 21)	Use (DHHS aims to prevent the use, not abuse, of alcohol and other drugs by youth)
Responsible use	Use (since there is risk associated with all use)
Drunk driving (because a person does not have to be drunk to be impaired)	Alcohol-impaired driving
Accidents when referring to alcohol and other drug use	Crashes (since the term "accident" suggests the event could not have been avoided)

In referring to alcohol as a drug, reduction-of-consumption proponents are technically correct. Pharmacologically "any substance that by its chemical nature alters structure or function in the living organism is a drug. . . . Pharmacological effects are exerted by foods, vitamins, hormones, microbial metabolites, plants, snake venoms, stings, products of decay, air pollutants, pesticides, minerals, synthetic chemicals, virtually all foreign materials (very few are completely inert), and many materials normally in the body" (Modell, 1967, p. 346).[3] However, their intent appears to be to stigmatize alcohol by associating it with illicit drugs. This is frequently accomplished by discussing alcohol in the same paragraph with crack cocaine and other illicit drugs. Often the effort is more direct. The Maine State Department of Education (n.d.) states, "The term 'alcohol/drug' is used to emphasize that alcohol is a mind-altering drug needing equal consideration with all other mind-altering drugs," the Florida Department of Education refers to alcohol as a harmful drug (Morton, 1990, p. 6), Oregon's Department (Mielke and Holstedt, 1991, p. 472) states unequivocally that wine coolers are illegal drugs, and Georgia's Department (Georgia Department of Education, n.d., p. 15) contends, without any qualification, that alcohol is harmful to the body. A poster distributed by the New York State Division of Alcoholism and Alcohol Abuse (n.d.) poses in large upper-case letters the question "DO YOU USE DRUGS?" above a picture of a bottle of beer; at the bottom it asserts: "More people get into trouble with alcohol than any other drug. Beer contains alcohol." Another poster warns in large letters above a bottle of a wine cooler "Don't be fooled"; below it warns in large letters "This is a drug" (New York State Division of Alcoholism and Alcohol Abuse, n.d.).

An OSAP publication (Office for Substance Abuse Prevention, 1987, p. 11) describes alcohol as a poison and implies that drinking might lead to death. Similarly, the State Education Department of New York (n.d., p. 30) defines alcohol as toxic. Another OSAP publication (1988, p. 16) asserts that the effects of alcohol—no level or degree of usage indicated—are that "[b]rain cells are altered and may die. Memory formation is blocked. . . . In men hormone levels change, causing lower sex drive and enlarged breasts. Women's menstrual cycles become irregular, and their ovaries malfunction. Deterioration of the heart muscle can occur." As indicated earlier, the WCTU similarly argued that alcohol can weaken the heart. However, it clearly specified its assertion that this may occur slowly "When alcohol is constantly [presumably it meant continually] used." OSAP provides no such qualifier. The same OSAP publication (p.17) presents "Four Basic Stages of Alcohol and Other Drug Use," according to which, in stage four, "Blackouts and overdosing are more common, family life is a disaster, and crime may be becoming a way of life." The presentation clearly implies a natural, if not inexorable, progression through the stages to a life of disaster, an assertion traditionally made by temperance writers.

OSAP also uses religion in its efforts to stigmatize alcohol. For example, it distributes a pamphlet showing a sword cutting through an alcohol bottle along with the admonition "The Word of God speaks with striking forcefulness against the evil of drinking. The truth concerning this evil cannot be ignored or escaped" (Office for Substance Abuse Prevention, 1993, p. 3). While this sounds very much like something Mary Hunt or a temperance minister might have written, they did not have the benefit of tax revenues to proselytize their religious beliefs.

REDUCTION-OF-CONSUMPTION EDUCATION REJECTS MODERATION

In its *Drug Prevention Education: A Guide to Selection and Implementation*, the U.S. Department of Education (1988, pp. 10–11) asserts that curricular materials should present "a clear and consistent message that the use of alcohol, tobacco, and other illicit drugs is unhealthy [sic] and harmful" and warns that in some curricula that message "is lost altogether as publishers strive to balance conflicting views." Educators selecting a curriculum are also specifically warned:

Curricula which advocate "*responsible use*" of drugs should be rejected. Such curricula tend to foster a belief that some illicit drugs, especially marijuana, are not particularly harmful if used in moderation. Yet we know from research that marijuana and other drugs, including alcohol and tobacco, can have devastating effects, especially on developing bodies. While today's curricula seldom urge "responsible use" in the same explicit fashion as those marketed in the 1970s, consumers should be alert to curricula which rely even implicitly on camouflaged versions of this theory.

For example, pay attention if a curriculum tells students that drugs themselves are neither good nor bad, but that *how* they are used is the most important factor.

Another warning sign is the "some believe this . . . while others believe that" approach which avoids being "judgmental" about drugs. Phrases like "research is inconclusive" or "not enough is known to make a judgment" about the effects of drugs are red flags. There is a wealth of conclusive research about the harmful effects of drugs, and curricula should not waffle on this point. Any curriculum which contains unclear messages about using dangerous substances should be rejected. (U. S. Department of Education, 1988, pp. 10–11, ellipses and emphasis in original)

Alcohol: the Gateway Drug, New York State's curriculum guide for kindergarten through twelfth grade, is consistent with federal policy:

Associated with the continued public acceptance of alcohol as a benign substance rather than a mind-altering, addictive drug is the concept of "responsible drinking."

While responsible drinking programs recognize that youth under the legal possession age are faced with choices about alcohol use, the strategy automatically presumes that the "normal" choice will be use. The message that non-use is the choice strongly preferred by society for young people is often overlooked, as is the fact that laws must be broken for young people to use alcohol except under parental supervision. The strategy also implies that responsible use is a way to prevent alcohol problems. The word "responsible" itself suggests that some "irresponsibility" is at the root of alcohol problems, something we *know* is inaccurate. Non-use is the only sure way to prevent alcohol problems. (New York State Division of Alcoholism and Alcohol Abuse, n.d., p. 2, emphasis in original)

The idea that people can use alcohol in moderation is even described by some reduction-of-control writers as a deadly message that educators must avoid (Horton, 1989), a view held by Mary Hunt and other Scientific Temperance Instruction promoters.

REDUCTION-OF-CONSUMPTION POLICIES AND PROHIBITIONISM: HOW DIFFERENT?

It should be noted that the beliefs as well as the policies commonly promoted by reduction-of-consumption advocates appear to be virtually identical to those of the Anti-Saloon League and the American Temperance League (now combined and known as the American Council on Alcohol Problems) and similar groups, a fact acknowledged by a leading control of consumption writer (Schmidt, 1985, p. 107). Consequently, it is difficult to differentiate between materials produced by such groups as the NIAAA and the American Council on Alcohol Problems or the National Temperance and Prohibition Council. For example, the American Council on Alcohol Problems asserts that "problems relating to alcohol and other drugs are in direct proportion to consumption. More consumers and higher per capita consumption produce increased problems . . ." and it advocates "activities aimed at reducing both the number of consumers of alcohol (and other drugs), and the per capita rate of consumption" (American Council on Alcohol Problems, n.d., p. 2). It takes pride in its role in

- Restoring "Age 21" laws for purchasing alcohol in all fifty states
- Mandating of warning labels on alcoholic beverage containers
- Increasing federal excise taxes on alcoholic beverages. (American Council on Alcohol Problems, n.d., p. 2)

This abstinence group also strongly promotes other reduction-of-consumption measures, such as strict controls on alcohol advertising and marketing practices, including a ban on TV ads and mandated warning labels on all ads and promotions (American Council on Alcohol Problems, n.d., p. 2).

The founder of the WCTU, Frances Willard, wrote in 1895 that "All the work we do is based on . . . the prohibition of the legalized sale of intoxicating liquors as beverages enacted by the town, county, state or nation. Whatever tends directly to this result, viz: restricted hours of sale, Sunday closing, prohibition of the sale to minors and drunkards, we . . . will strongly favor" (Willard, 1895, p. 43).

The National Temperance and Prohibition Council echoes the NIAAA in referring to alcohol as a drug and a poison (National Temperance and Prohibition Council, 1991, p. 1) and in its efforts "To emphasize the deceptiveness of the word 'abuse' [by] indicating the danger as being in alcohol and other drug *use*, not only its abuse" (National Temperance and Prohibition Council, n.d., p. 2, emphasis in original).

It has been noted that the mythmaking tactics of neo-prohibitionists resemble those of the prohibitionists:

Like their prohibitionist predecessors, they claim scientific legitimacy for their approach in the face of highly inconsistent research evidence (Heath, 1986, 1990), including compelling evidence that alcohol availability and consumption are not necessarily or mechanically linked (Mulford, Ledolter & Fitzgerald, 1992, 1993). They exaggerate the growth of alcohol abuser numbers. In its successive reports to Congress since 1971, the NIAAA has essentially doubled the alcoholic/problem drinker prevalence figures by changing its terminology and by changing its definition of the target population (Heath, 1990). They also exaggerate the financial cost of alcohol abuse (Heien & Pittman, 1993). Moreover, the claim that, because alcohol has been found associated with certain social problems, it therefore causes them. (Mulford, 1994, p. 519)

When neo-drys insist that alcohol is a drug and then demand "a totally drug-free environment in the school and community" (Horton, 1989, p. 39), are they calling for anything other than a return to prohibition?

After decades of propaganda by the WCTU and innumerable other temperance proselytizers, it is not surprising that many temperance beliefs and attitudes are now a part of our culture. The percentage of abstainers in the United States is, along with Ireland's, the highest among Western nations (Peele, 1989, p. 43). In a 1987 Gallup Poll, 17 percent of the Americans interviewed said they would favor a law forbidding the sale of alcoholic beverages throughout the nation (Room, 1991, p. 156). The neo-dry movement is a natural and understandable consequence of these facts.

The temperance movement appears to have had a strong appeal to authoritarian (Sinclair, 1962, ch. 2) and dogmatic (or closed minded) persons. Such individuals tend to accept simplistic solutions to complex problems. They are intolerant of ambiguity and tend to see issues in dichotomized terms (Hanson, 1967, ch. 2). The temperance movement defined individuals as either abstainers or drunkards; abstinence was good, drinking was bad. Moderation or responsible use was rejected. Alcohol itself was not defined as a substance that could be used or abused: it was a poison. Thus, "either a person was *for* the movement or was *for* its enemies, the Wets" (Bacon, 1970, p. 135, emphases in original).

The new temperance proponents of today similarly reject ambiguity and uncertainty. Recall that the U.S. Department of Education (1988, p. 11, emphasis in original), for example, asserts, "Curricula which advocate '*responsible use*' of drugs should be rejected." It similarly warns against curricula that teach that "drugs themselves are neither good nor bad." The complexity of real life must be denied so as not to send conflicting messages. Recall that "another warning sign [of an unacceptable curriculum] is the 'some believe this . . . while others believe that' approach which avoids being 'judgmental' about drugs. Phrases like 'research is inconclusive' or 'not enough is known to make a judgment' about the effects of drugs are red flags." Similarly, the WCTU never feared being judgmental about alcohol or its effects and was intolerant of mixed messages. Recall also that, like the WCTU, the Office for Substance Abuse Prevention (1987, p. 11) describes alcohol as a poison.

The temperance movement generally rejected both immigrants and their use of alcohol. It is ironic that the neo-temperance movement of today rejects the lessons that can be learned from the successful use of alcohol by many of those same immigrant groups.

THERE IS A BETTER WAY

For thousands of years a number of societies have used alcohol extensively with few problems. Most of their members have drunk alcohol daily since early childhood, consumed a variety of alcohol beverages, imbibed them in numerous settings, and yet have rarely abused the substance (Greeley et al., 1980, pp. 38–39; Lolli et al., 1958, p. xii; Unkovic et al., 1980, p. 171; Chafetz and Demone, 1962, pp. 84, 86–88; Snyder, 1958, pp. 113–140, 183–202; Glassner and Berg, 1985, pp. 94, 102, 104; Barnett, 1955) What accounts for the very successful use of alcohol by Italians, Jews, Greeks and many other peoples around the world?

First, such groups tend to view alcohol as a natural and normal part of life. Alcohol is seen as neither a poison nor a magic elixir capable of solving problems or conferring adulthood.

Second, there is no pressure for members of these groups to drink. Abstaining and drinking in moderation are both seen as equally valid and acceptable options.[4] However, the abuse of alcohol is strictly prohibited and is not tolerated under any circumstances.

Finally, young people learn at home how to drink in moderation from their parents who teach by good example (Blacker, 1966; Marshall, 1979; Robbins, 1979).

THE SOCIOCULTURAL APPROACH

The sociocultural approach to alcohol, based on the successful experience of Italians, Jews, Greeks and many other groups around the world, assumes that:

1. It is the misuse of alcohol, not alcohol itself, that is the source of drinking problems.
2. It is important to distinguish between alcohol use and abuse.
3. The misuse of alcohol can be reduced by educating individuals to make one of two decision:
   • one decision is to abstain;
   • the other decision is to drink responsibly.
4. Because many individuals will choose to drink alcohol, it is important that societal norms regarding what is acceptable and unacceptable behavior for those who choose to drink be clear and unambiguous.
5. People who are going to drink as adults should gradually learn how to drink. Preferably, this should occur first in the home from the parents and then be reinforced through formal education in schools.

From this perspective, it is essential that all attempts to stigmatize beverage alcohol as a "dirty drug" or a poison, as inherently harmful, or as a substance to be abhorred should be stopped. Stigmatizing alcohol may inadvertently trivialize the use of illegal drugs and thereby encourage their use. For example, attempts to stigmatize alcohol may create the false impression, especially among younger students, that parents who use alcohol in moderation are drug abusers thereby reversing the good example they project. A misguided effort to equate alcohol with illicit drugs is likely to be counterproductive.

Educational efforts should encourage moderate use of alcohol among those who choose to drink. Such efforts should present moderation in drinking rather than drinking *per se* as a sign of maturity (Wilkinson, 1970, p. 105).

Alcohol can confer neither adulthood nor masculinity. Unfortunately, a common "cause of trouble is the belief that an ability to 'hold one's liquor' is a sign of manliness; in many circles heavy drinking is equated with masculinity. This belief encourages the drinking of large amounts of alcohol and promotes drunkenness. Because of this linkage of drinking with masculinity, some adolescents and young men (and perhaps older men as well) choose this readily available and generally approved way of demonstrating to themselves and others that they 'really are men'" (Plaut, 1967, p. 130).

It is important that educational efforts present moderate drinking and abstinence as equally acceptable or appropriate choices, and just as those who choose to drink should not force alcohol on abstainers, "those who choose not to drink alcohol should not attempt to impose that decision or the values surrounding the decision on others" (Education Commission of the States, n.d., p. 4).

Consistent with the sociocultural view, Cisin (1978, p. 154) has observed:

In our roles as parents and educators, we have responsibility for the socialization of our children, a responsibility for preparing them for life in the world. Part of our job is teaching children how to handle dangerous activities like driving, swimming, drinking, and sex. We behave toward our children as though there were really two different kinds of dangerous activities. Driving and swimming fall into the first type: we carefully teach our children that these are dangerous activities, and we deliberately set out to be sure that they know there is a right way and a wrong way to participate in these activities.

On the other hand, when we look at the other kind of dangerous activities, exemplified by drinking and sex, we seem to know only one word: 'Don't.' We do not bother to say there is a right way and there is a wrong way; we just say 'Don't!' We do not really want to produce abstainers; we have the illusion that they will follow our advice and be abstainers (in the case of sex, until marriage; and in the case of alcohol, until maturity) until they reach the magic age at which they can handle these activities. But as to the rights and wrongs of handling it when the great day comes, we choose to keep them in the dark. Now this is sheer hypocrisy. We are slowly awakening to the fact that we owe our children sex education in the home and in the school—education not dominated by the antisex league. We should be brave enough to tell them the truth; that drinking is normal behavior in the society, that moderate drinking need not lead to abuse; that drinking can be done in an appropriate civilized way without shame and guilt. Perhaps greater socialization in the direction of moderate drinking is part of the program we need for prevention of alcohol problems in the future.

GUIDELINES FOR RESPONSIBLE ALCOHOL USE

The Education Commission of the States Task Force on Responsible Decisions About Alcohol (n.d., p. 4) identified guidelines for the responsible use of alcohol:

A. Situational Responsibilities

1. Alcohol should not be the main focus of a gathering. Food and recreational activities should be available.
2. In serving beverage alcohol, measure correctly and do not push drinks.
3. Recognize the decision of others to drink or not to drink. Have beverages to accommodate both.
4. Recognize drunkenness as unacceptable behavior.
5. Recognize alcohol problems in yourself and others. Try to get or offer help.
6. Understand your own decision regarding the use of beverage alcohol.
7. Use alcohol in a relaxed setting and avoid drinking alone.
8. Recognize and make plans to promote the concepts of responsibility for the health and safety of others.

B. Health Responsibilities

1. Stay within your limit when using beverage alcohol.
2. Recognize alcohol as a drug, don't combine its use with other drugs. It may combine unfavorably.
3. Recognize that alcohol can not solve problems.
4. Recognize that for those who suffer from the disease alcoholism, the most responsible decision is to abstain.

C. Safety Responsibilities

1. Avoid performing complex tasks such as driving a car, operating machinery or engaging in physical activities while under the influence of alcohol.
2. Avoid riding with a driver who is under the influence.
3. Recognize that your behaviors and attitudes influence others, especially children.

At about the same time, the National Institute on Alcoholism and Alcohol Abuse issued a set of guidelines to assist teachers in educating about alcohol:

1. Alcohol is a drug that can cause positive and negative social, psychological, and physical effects.
2. The responsible use of alcohol can be socially, psychologically, and physically beneficial.
3. To drink or not to drink should be a personal decision. However, those who drink have a responsibility not to damage themselves or society.
4. People who drink should respect the decision of those who do not drink.
5. People who serve alcoholic beverages should not push drinks on others, in an effort to contribute to a healthy drinking environment.
6. Intoxication is not responsible drinking.
7. There is a direct link between responsible attitudes toward drinking and the alleviation of the problem of alcoholism. (Miller, 1982, p. 43)

The U.S. Jaycees developed a program to encourage responsible consumption of alcohol known as Operation THRESHOLD. That program also established guidelines for responsible use:

1. Drinks are to be sipped.
2. Food is to be consumed before or during the consumption of beverage alcohol.
3. Drinking is to be undertaken in a relaxed, comfortable setting.
4. Knowledge of one's limit, and the ability to stick to it, are important.
5. Drunkenness is not humorous, or masculine, and is not to be tolerated.
6. The decision of those who choose not to drink is to be respected.
7. One drink an hour— as a rule of thumb only—is not that unrealistic.
8. Drinking is not to be the primary activity, it is only an adjunct. (Dolan, 1976, p. 24)

It has been suggested that responsible use of alcohol would mean, for example, not drinking if a person is alcoholic, ill, taking certain medications, or serving as a designated driver. It would also mean never becoming drunk and never having to feel sorry for what has happened as a result of consuming alcohol (Hanson and Engs, 1994, p. 177). Practical and specific guidelines for responsible drinking include:

1. Know your limit. If you do not already know how much alcohol you can handle without losing control, try it out one time at home, with your parents or roommate present. Explain to them what you are attempting to learn. Most people find that taking no more than a drink and a half per hour will keep them in control of the situation and avoid drunkenness.

2. Eat food while you drink. It is particularly good to eat high protein foods such as cheese and peanuts, which help to slow the absorption of alcohol into the circulatory system.

3. Sip your drink. If you gulp a drink for the effect that it produces, you are losing a pleasure of drinking, namely savoring the taste and aroma. This is particularly true of wine.

4. Accept a drink only when you really want one. If someone tries to force a drink on you, ask for an alternative beverage.

5. Cultivate taste. Choose quality rather than quantity. Learn the names of fine wines, whiskeys, and beers and learn which beverages taste best with various foods.

6. Skip a drink occasionally. At parties, have a nonalcoholic drink between alcoholic ones, to keep your blood alcohol concentration down. Also, space out your alcoholic drinks to maintain a low blood alcohol concentration.

7. If you must drive home after drinking, have your drink(s) before or with dinner rather than afterward. This permits time for the alcohol to be absorbed slowly into the circulatory system and burned up. Consume no more than one drink per hour.

8. Beware of unfamiliar drinks. Drinks such as zombies and other fruit and rum drinks can be deceiving because the degree of alcohol is not always detectable by taste.

9. Make sure that alcohol improves social relationships rather than impairs them. Serve alcohol as an adjunct to an activity rather than as the primary focus.

10. Appoint a designated driver. Have someone available who will not be drinking and will drive others home.

11. Use alcohol cautiously in connection with prescription or over-the-counter-drugs. If in any doubt, consult your physician or pharmacist regarding possible negative drug interactions.

12. Respect the rights of those who do not wish to drink. It is inconsiderate and rude to attempt to get people to drink if they do not wish to do so. They may abstain for religious or medical reasons, because they are recovering alcoholics, or just because they don't like the taste of alcohol or the effect it has on them. In any case, the reason is their business and their choice not to drink should be respected.

13. Avoid drinking alcohol (especially mixed drinks) on an empty stomach on hot days. This can produce hypoglycemia, leading to dizziness, weakness, and mood changes.

14. Avoid heavy drinking while pregnant. Research appears to suggest that heavy drinking among pregnant women may cause fetal alcohol syndrome. (Hanson and Engs, 1994, pp. 177–178)

Those who serve alcohol to their guests have an important role to play in promoting moderate consumption for those who choose to drink. Guidelines for responsible hosting include:

1. Pass the drinks. Serve drinks at regular, reasonable intervals along with plenty of nonalcoholic beverages. A schedule of one alcoholic drink per hour is a good guide.

2. Have a responsible bartender. If you plan to have a friend act as bartender, make sure that the person is not a drink pusher.

3. Don't serve doubles. Many people count and pace their drinks. If you serve doubles, they will be drinking twice as much as they intended.

4. Push snacks. Make sure that people are eating along with drinking.

5. Don't push the drinks. Let the glass become empty before you offer a refill.

6. Be sure to serve nonalcoholic beverages also. Remember that one out of five college students chooses not to drink. Make sure that you have a reasonable selection of appealing nonalcoholic drinks to serve.
7. End the party properly. Decide, in advance, when you want your party to end. Before that time, stop serving alcohol and offer coffee and a substantial snack. This provides some non-drinking time before your guests leave. (Hanson and Engs, 1994, p. 178)

A responsible decision might be not to drink if any two of the following applies to the individual:

1. Gulps drinks for the effect that rapid drinking produces.
2. Starts the day with a drink.
3. Drinks alone to escape from reality, boredom, loneliness, or anger.
4. Frequently gets intoxicated.
5. Drinks to relieve a hangover.
6. Loses time from school or work because of drinking.
7. Drinks to lose shyness or build self-confidence.
8. Drinking adversely affects reputation.
9. Drinks to escape from worries.
10. Bothered if someone suggests he or she might drink too much.
11. Takes a drink in order to face a situation.
12. Experiences financial problems because of buying alcohol.
13. Has lost friends since beginning to drink.
14. Hangs-around with a group that drinks a lot.
15. Drinks more than friends do.
16. Drinks until the bottle is empty.
17. Has had a loss of memory from drinking.
18. Has ended up in jail or hospital as a result of driving while intoxicated.
19. Gets annoyed with lectures or classes on drinking.
20. Thinks they have a problem with drinking. (adapted from Hanson and Engs, 1994, pp. 178–179)

We must have the courage and integrity to stop being educational ostriches. First, we must start with a:

realistic acceptance of certain facts. Alcohol is widely available and consumed in American society and teen-agers, as well as adults, must choose if, how and under what circumstances they will or will not drink. In a democratic society of which alcohol is a part, the only realistic, practical hope is that people will make choices about alcohol consumption that reduce their risk of alcohol-related problems. Alcohol education efforts should be focused on enabling people to adopt and maintain those low-risk choices.
   A definition of low-risk choices . . . includes 1) the choice to abstain and for persons who do drink 2) the choice of a quantity and frequency of alcohol consumption that presents little, if any, risk for developing alcohol-related problems. (Thompson et al., 1984, p. 80)

Most college students drink and most typically drink in moderation. However, collegians drink within a set of norms differing from those in the larger society. Furthermore, being away from home for the first time may result in experimentation with excessive drinking. During the freshman year, in particular, students may test their limits by staying up late, sleeping late, eating too much of the wrong foods, and similar excessive behaviors. Haines (1983, p. 3) observed that "It is precisely for these reasons that college students are an ideal population at an opportune stage of development to be taught healthy drinking practices. As early as 1976 *The Whole College Catalog About Drinking* listed, ' . . . communicate what constitutes safe drinking practices for those who choose to drink' among its four fundamental goals of alcohol abuse prevention (DHEW, 1976)" (Haines, 1983, p. 3).

We have clearly learned much about how to achieve this from the successful alcohol experience of the American colonists as well as the Italians, Greeks, Jews and many others from which the current sociocultural model has emerged. But the prohibitionist impulse is also alive and well today in the reduction-of-consumption approach to alcohol. This leads us to consider the current nature of alcohol education.

CONTEMPORARY ALCOHOL EDUCATION

Mary Hunt's long and concerted efforts clearly had an enormous impact on the nature of alcohol education, which all 50 states now legally mandate (Horton, 1989, p. 38). Another event of major importance was the rise of drug education, beginning in the mid-1960s. This event was significant because education about alcohol (a legal substance) became a part of education about illicit drugs. To this day, alcohol is typically treated as a component in drug education courses. More importantly, the educational treatment given to alcohol is dominated by that given to illegal drugs.

In the 1960s, LSD (lysergic acid diethylamide), marijuana, methaqualone, amphetamines, and barbiturates became household terms as an epidemic of highly visible and well publicized drug use occurred among middle class young people (Inciardi, 1986, p. 188). Timothy Leary, a well-known Harvard University psychologist, actively promoted the use of illegal drugs to enhance self-understanding and express personal freedom from societal restraints on behavior. By the mid-1960s, the American people became alarmed as "the use of widely known illicit drugs seemed to have spread beyond the confines of the inner cities and became more evident in all areas of the country" (Goldberg and Meyers, 1980, p. 126). Increasingly, middle-class Americans felt threatened by drugs and insisted that something be done and be done quickly.

Between 1968 and 1973, the National Institute of Mental Health produced and distributed over 22 million antidrug pamphlets (Zinberg, 1984). In 1970, the president of the United States asserted that drug abuse education, as a preventive measure of the highest national priority, must reach all publicly educated children from kindergarten through the twelfth grade (Einstein et al., 1971, pp. 324–325). Subsequently, federal and state expenditures for drug education, information, and training increased dramatically and an enormous bureaucracy for the delivery of drug education was developed (Hanson, 1980, p. 251). By the early 1970s, most of the 17,000 school districts across the United States had implemented drug education instruction (Zinberg, 1984, p. 205).

Just as the temperance writers assumed that teaching the evils of alcohol in schools would frighten students into abstinence, it was now believed that teaching the evils of drugs would frighten young people into avoiding them. Drug education appeared to be operating in the long shadow of Mary Hunt.

While Mary Hunt had to contend with the Committee of Fifty, the new drug educators had their commissions, councils, and other critics with which to deal. Some observers argued that drug education not only failed to prevent or reduce drug use, it might actually stimulate interest in drug experimentation and use. Indeed, illegal drug use continued to escalate despite school programs (Goldberg and Meyers, 1980, p. 133; Kallmeyer, 1980, p. 251).

The Shafer Commission determined in 1973 that much of the information in drug education programs was inaccurate (Mahaffey, 1988, p. 14). The National Coordinating Council on Drug Education reviewed 220 drug education films and found that "33% of the films were so inaccurate or distorted as to be totally unacceptable, 50% were not suited for general audiences unless a skilled instructor was present, and only 16% were scientifically and conceptually acceptable" (Zinberg, 1984, p. 205). In the same year, the National Commission on Marijuana and Drug Abuse called for "a moratorium on the production and distribution of new drug information materials until standards for accuracy could be developed and existing materials analyzed" (Goldberg and Meyers, 1980, p. 130). It recognized the lack of knowledge regarding the impact of drug education and recommended a moratorium on all drug education programs in the schools, at least until existing programs could be evaluated. It asserted that "no drug education program in this country, or elsewhere, has proven sufficiently successful to warrant our recommending it," and speculated that "the avalanche of drug education in recent years has been counterproductive," and may have stimulated rebellion or simply raised interest in the forbidden (National Commission on Marijuana and Drug Abuse, 1973, pp. 356–357).

In 1977, the Cabinet Committee on Drug Abuse Prevention, Treatment and Rehabilitation concluded that young people would continue to experiment with illicit drugs as a natural part of growing up. Therefore, it recommended that drug education efforts be "primarily focused on moderating the effects of drug taking." The new goal recommended by the committee was: "educate to prevent harmful use" (Goldberg and Meyers, 1980, p. 132). However, it would appear that few heeded the recommendation. That very year, the federal government adopted the reduction-of-consumption policy regarding alcohol and within a few years the "Just Say No" policy was in effect regarding both alcohol and drugs. Drug-free schools, zero tolerance, and similar phrases became household terms.

THE DRUG-FREE SCHOOLS AND COMMUNITIES ACT

The U.S. Department of Education administers the Drug-Free Schools and Communities Act, which attempts to prevent alcohol and drug abuse problems in primary schools, secondary schools, and colleges.[5] It is the federal government's largest school-based alcohol and drug abuse prevention program, recently funded at well over one-half billion dollars per year (Government Information Services, 1991, p. B-7). This money funds a wide range of programs:

1. Grants to states, largely to fund local efforts to improve anti-drug abuse education, prevention, early intervention and rehabilitation referral programs.
2. Grants for colleges and universities (administered through the Fund for the Improvement of Postsecondary Education) to develop, implement, operate and improve drug education for college students.
3. Grants to provide drug and alcohol abuse education and prevention services for Native Americans enrolled in elementary and secondary schools funded by the Bureau of Indian Affairs.
4. Grants to Native Hawaiian organizations to plan, conduct and administer alcohol and drug education and prevention programs.
5. Grants to support five Department of Education regional centers to:
   • train school teams to assess drug and alcohol abuse programs;
   • assist State Educational Agencies in coordinating and strengthening alcohol and drug abuse education and prevention programs;
   • assist local educational agencies and institutions of higher education in developing teacher training programs; and
   • evaluate and disseminate information on effective substance abuse education and prevention strategies/programs.
6. Grants to provide for the training of school teachers and administrators regarding drug and alcohol abuse prevention and education.
7. Grants to provide for the training of counselors, psychologists, nurses and social workers who administer drug and alcohol abuse prevention, counseling or referral services to schools.
8. Grants to fund the development of materials for alcohol abuse education targeting teachers working in grades five through eight.
9. Grants to provide financial assistance to schools demonstrating a high-risk need for additional resources in combating drug and alcohol abuse.
10. Grants to fund Federal activities supporting model development, dissemination, technical assistance, and curriculum development activities. The Department of Education supports a number of projects and positions in this category including:
    • the staff of the Division of Drug-Free Schools and Communities in the Office of Elementary and Secondary education,
    • drug prevention videotapes for distribution to elementary and secondary schools,
    • a "Very Special Arts Program" at the Kennedy Center,
    • a quarterly newsletter, *The Challenge*,
    • the National Clearinghouse for Alcohol and Drug Information
    • a publication, *Schools Without Drugs*, to supply assistance to schools and communities about developing drug and alcohol abuse prevention programs,
    • a handbook, *Growing Up Drug-Free: A Parent's Guide to Prevention*,
    • lesson plans and activities for teachers, *Learning to Live Drug-Free: A Curriculum Model for Prevention*,
    • activities and programs that are jointly developed by the Office of Educational Research and Improvement, such as: the Drug-Free School Recognition

Program, Network of Drug-Free Colleges, Early Childhood Education Drug Prevention Materials, and the *Drug Prevention Curricula Guide,*
- studies on the Department of Education's drug prevention efforts supported by the Planning and Evaluation Services, and
- programs at other Federal Agencies. (U. S. Department of Education, 1993, pp. 1–8)

Higher education was clearly not immune from this legislation. In 1986, Congress authorized monies for a Fund for the Improvement of Postsecondary Education program which provides grants to colleges and universities for alcohol and drug education and prevention programs. Congress also passed legislation requiring colleges and universities to have alcohol and drug education programs in place in order to qualify for federal financial aid monies (DeLoughry, 1989a, p. A1; 1989b, p. A15; 1989c, p. A30; Palmer, 1986, p. A1). Two years later, Congress passed legislation requiring students receiving federal financial aid to sign an affidavit stating that they do not use illegal drugs, defined as including alcohol if they are under 21 years of age (Wilson and Cordes, 1988, p. A16) even when legal to do so. The federal government has also threatened to conduct random on-site investigations of college students receiving federal financial aid to determine if they are using illegal drugs (Jaschik, 1989, p. A1).

In 1989, the president signed into law the Drug Free Schools and Communities Act Amendments,which require that each and every institution of higher education receiving any federal funds adopt and implement an alcohol and drug prevention program. All such colleges and universities are required to notify every student and employee annually of:

1. Standards of conduct that clearly prohibit, at a minimum, the unlawful possession, use, or distribution of illicit drugs or alcohol by students and employees on [their] property or as part of any of [their] activities.
2. The applicable legal sanctions under local, state, or federal law for the unlawful possession or distribution of illicit drugs or alcohol.
3. The health risks associated with the use of illicit drugs and the abuse of alcohol.
4. Any drug or alcohol counseling, treatment, or rehabilitation programs available to employees or students.
5. A clear statement that the IHE [institution of higher education] will impose disciplinary sanctions on students and employees consistent with local, state, or federal law, and a description of those sanction, up to and including expulsion or termination of employment and referral for prosecution for violations of the standards of conduct required by paragraph (a)(1) of this section. (Drug Free Schools and Campus Rules, 34CFR86.100)

Less than two months before the law went into effect, the Department of Education issued regulations for distributing the mandated information. It decided that while the phrase "in writing" did not appear in the law, institutions *must* distribute the required materials in writing to each student and employee and that merely making them available to everyone would not be legally acceptable (Palmer et al., 1992, p. 31).

The shadow of Mary Hunt has proven to be very long and very dark.

ISSUES IN DEVELOPING CURRICULA

In addition to the reduction-of-consumption versus responsible use debate, basic issues faced in developing an alcohol education program include the objectives, the target group, the teaching personnel, and the content and methods to be employed.

Objectives

Objectives of alcohol education are typically categorized as being cognitive (beliefs), affective (attitudes and feelings), and behavioral (actions). Ironically, while most people would probably agree that the most important objectives would be behavioral, alcohol curricula typically focus primarily on cognitive objectives, moderately on affective objectives, and concentrate the least on behavioral objectives.

It is important to recognize that teaching alcohol knowledge may have little, if any, impact on either attitudes on behavior regarding alcohol. Changing attitudes has little, if any, impact on actual behavior (Staulcup, 1980, p. 103). Objectives can also be short- or long-range in nature; and while it is long range objectives that are typically seen as being of greater importance, it is usually short range effects that are identified and measured. Because the effects of education tend to decay or disappear over time, the identification of educational effects in the short run tends to magnify or exaggerate the apparent value of educational programs.

Among the objectives of alcohol education, the following are often identified:

1. to maintain total abstinence;
2. to delay the age at which consumption of alcohol begins;
3. to maintain current quantity or frequency levels of alcohol consumption;
4. to reduce the quantity or frequency of alcohol consumption;
5. to bring about a cessation of drinking;
6. to reduce or eliminate high-risk drinking behaviors (driving while intoxicated, riding with intoxicated drivers, etc.);
7. to increase accurate knowledge about alcohol;
8. to change attitudes about alcohol;[6]
9. to bring about informed decision-making about alcohol;
10. to assist students' emotional maturity and stability so as to reduce motivation to use alcohol;
11. to bring about values clarification;
12. to develop students' ability to resist peer pressure to drink; and
13. to encourage behaviors that might be adopted as alternatives to alcohol use

Objectives are often confusing to those not familiar with the curriculum in question. For example, the objective of teaching "responsible decisions regarding alcohol" often really means the objective of teaching students to decide not to drink. Similarly, "positive attitudes" often means negative attitudes toward alcohol and alcohol use (Cooper, 1989, p. 8).

Unfortunately it has been noted that:

The goal of abstinence is sometimes "concealed" in vaguely enunciated program goal statements. Undefined value-laden terms, which are subject to multiple interpretations, such as "healthy attitudes," "rational choice," "positive self concept," "proper behavior toward drugs," "values clarified individual," and the like, add further to the confusion. It is only upon closer scrutiny of their respective methodologies and evaluation criteria that the goal of abstinence is exposed. (Chng, 1981, p. 15)

While changes in knowledge and attitudes may have no impact on behavior, the same is also true of changes in values, self-concept, emotional security, self-awareness and other variables that alcohol education often attempts to manipulate. However, alcohol educators typically consider changes in such variables to constitute success.

In all cases objectives should be explicit, consistent with other objectives of the larger educational framework and understood by those charged with achieving them. Clearly, specifying the objectives of alcohol education is especially important when evaluation of its effectiveness is to be conducted. It is not acceptable for educational activities to be conducted unless there are objectives either in the short-term or long-term. In particular, health education should attempt to achieve significant shifts in knowledge, attitudes and, ultimately, behavior. Consequently, the future initiatives in this field should be devised with such specific and explicit aims in mind. Evaluational strategies should also be designed to examine whether such key variables are influenced, and if so in which direction and to what degree (Bagnall and Plant, 1987, p. 420).

Target Groups

The potential target groups of a drug prevention education program are typically categorized as either the general public or as subgroups of the general public. Subgroups are sometimes identified on the basis of social role, such as parents, physicians, police, students, politicians, clergy, and so on. Subgroups can also be identified according to stage of intervention. Such stages are usually categorized as primary, secondary, and tertiary. Primary prevention efforts occur when most or all of the individuals in the target group are abstainers. Secondary prevention efforts occur when many in the target group have experimented with alcohol or regularly use alcohol, while tertiary prevention efforts occur when most or all in the groups do experience, or have experienced, some difficulty as a result of drinking. A common example of tertiary prevention would be classes for drivers convicted for driving while under the influence of alcohol (Fischer, 1990, p. 36).

There is evidence that alcohol education should be introduced in early childhood while beliefs, attitudes, and behavior patterns are in their formulative period

(Bradley, 1988, p. 99; Tricker, 1985, p. 3; Wilusz and Parker, 1982, p. 14). Most alcohol education programs exist in schools, and while school students can be viewed as a single target population, they clearly are not a homogeneous group. The educational needs of kindergartners are different from those of college seniors, just as the needs of abstainers differ from those of chronic alcohol abusers (Brown, 1990, p. 6).

The fact that most alcohol education programs occur in schools is understandable. Students in school constitute captive audiences of relatively young and impressionable individuals. On the other hand, attendance by most nonschool groups is voluntary. Programs for such groups also typically require physical facilities, trained staff, promotional activities, and money. The cost of programs for mass media use tends to be very high. As a consequence of these problems there are relatively few drug education programs for the nonschool population.

Evidence also suggests that a school program on alcohol education should ideally be part of a total community effort since students are also affected by the environment outside school. What is learned in school can then be reinforced (Benard, 1986, p. 3; Flanigan, 1987, pp. 11–12; Durrell and Bukoski, 1985, p. 379; Johnson et al., 1988, p. 584).

Teaching Personnel

While classroom teachers usually present alcohol education programs, health professionals, law enforcement officers, recovering alcoholics, and student volunteers are frequently used (Rapaport et al., 1994, p. 137; Lobello et al., 1988, p. 68; Glassford et al., 1991, pp. 66–67; Jensen et al., 1989, p. 241). It is often asserted that whoever presents a drug prevention program should ideally be someone students like and trust, who knows and will present relevant facts and materials accurately, and who is relaxed and comfortable teaching the subject.

Content and Method

There is general agreement today that alcohol education should be comprehensive and should focus not only on the physiological and pharmacological aspects of alcohol use and abuse, but also on the psychological and emotional, legal, social, economic, political, and moral implications of alcohol use and abuse. While alcohol education has traditionally been located in health and physical education courses, some authorities argue that it should also be infused into other parts of the curriculum.

An area of major concern to alcohol educators involves the methods to be used in achieving their objectives. Possible methods include the following:

1. Negative reinforcement—the negative reinforcement or "scare tactic" approach asserts that undesirable consequences (illness, emotional disturbance, death, etc.) can result from the use of alcohol. The basic assumption is that fear of consequences will prevent use. (Stainback and Rogers, 1983, p. 393)

2. Logic—the logical argument approach utilizes the presentation of facts which students can use in making personal decisions regarding alcohol use. The presentation can be either one-sided or two-sided. If one-sided, it may resemble the scare approach. The logical argument approach tends to assume that individuals are logical and rational decision makers regarding their own behavior. (Howe, 1989, p. 4)

3. Authority—the authoritative source approach uses traditional experts (medical personnel, law enforcement officers, scholars, etc.) or experiential experts (former abusers or recovering alcoholics) to present facts and/or opinions on alcohol abuse. It is assumed that such authorities enjoy a higher level of credibility than the classroom teacher. This approach may or may not utilize scare tactics. (Clayton et al., 1991, p. 296)

4. Self-examination and values clarification—self-examination and values clarification attempts to involve students in examining their values, beliefs, and feelings regarding themselves, their lives, and the role of alcohol. This approach assumes that students must come to know themselves and their values in order to make informed decisions regarding alcohol. (Chng, 1980, p. 119)

5. Peers—the peer approach utilizes students to lead (or aid in) discussions or other instructional activities with other students. With training, students leaders can assume the role of teacher. Alternatively, the group may act as a team in exploring the subject. It is assumed that students are strongly influenced by peer pressure and expectation. It also assumes that increasing students' responsibility for their own learning may increase their motivation to learn. (May, 1993, p. 197; Collins, 1980, pp. iv–vii; Carpenter, 1981; Kuehn, 1991, p. 72)

6. Alternatives—the alternatives approach seeks to introduce students to alternative activities in order to reduce or eliminate their desire either to become drinkers, or to maintain their consumption of alcohol. It is assumed that individuals crave "highs" and that "natural highs" found in sports or other activities will be perceived as acceptable substitutes for alcohol intoxication. (Moskowitz et al., 1983; Malvin et al., 1985)

7. Coping skills—the psychological and social coping skills development approach attempts to achieve its objective through role-playing exercises or any of a diversity of other techniques. It assumes that people who have a broad repertoire of acceptable ways for coping with stressful personal feelings and social situations are less likely to use alcohol in dealing with stress. (Horan and Williams, 1982, pp. 349–350)

8. Refusal skills—the refusal skills approach attempts to teach students practical techniques to avoid social pressures to drink (or to drink more) and assumes that the individuals receiving the training wish to abstain or to drink less than others might want them to consume. (Duryea, 1983, pp. 250–251; George, 1986, p. 4)

Alcohol education has relied (and continues to rely) heavily on conveying knowledge about the substance and its effects. This is true even in programs commonly described as emphasizing decision-making, values clarification, refusal skills, etc. It has been suggested by some that:

Many programs cling to information based materials as the "meat" of their curriculum because it presents discrete, testable information, easily and willingly learned by students, which gives program planners confidence in the fact that they have *taught* something and that the *something they have taught* will be evident in post test data. Such a curriculum, then, speaks to the insecurity that educators often feel in the preparation and implementation of drug programs. Most planners and evaluators do subscribe to the idea that some amount

of information about the specific effects of certain drugs is beneficial. The question lies in
the amount and specificity of information, and the difficulty lies in programs which present
this information as necessary and sufficient for prevention of use. (Argentos, 1991, p. 3,
emphases in original; also see Fullerton, 1983, pp. 9–11)

Regardless of the possible motives, the goal of increasing knowledge or
information is at least implicitly based on the commonly accepted knowledge-
attitude-behavior model of prevention, which is the most widely accepted model
of alcohol education (Andrews, 1987, pp. 86–87). It is assumed that changing or
increasing knowledge will change attitudes, which, in turn, will change behavior (Camacho, 1987, p. 18). The causal sequence is conceptualized as:
knowledge—>attitude—>behavior. Four submodels have been suggested:

1. knowledge change leads to behavior change,
2. attitude change leads to behavior change,
3. knowledge change leads to attitude change, which in turn, leads to behavior change,
4. behavioral change leads to attitudinal change, which, in turn reinforces or produces
   further behavior change. (Goodstadt and Caleekal-John, 1984, p. 723)

However, over 60 years ago, Richard La Piere collected evidence suggesting that
this model might be deficient by finding gross inconsistencies between attitudes
and actions. In his classic study, La Piere (1934) traveled across the United States
with a young Chinese couple and found that out of 251 separate transactions for
accommodation, they were refused service only once. However, six months later
La Piere sent a questionnaire to each of the establishments they had visited asking
if Chinese were acceptable as guests. Only one of those responding (128 of 251)
indicated that Chinese would be served, nine were uncertain, while all the rest
(92%) asserted that Chinese would be refused service. Since that time voluminous
evidence has mounted indicating discontinuities between attitudes and behaviors,
and between knowledge and behavior (Liska, 1975; Deutscher, 1973; Fischer,
1990; Butler, 1982, p. 606; Gonzalez, 1982, p. 2; Stolberg, 1987; Andrews, 1987,
p. 88; Dupont and Jason, 1984, pp. 373–374; Goodstadt, 1985, p. 85; Polish et al.,
1984, p. 23). Nevertheless, the knowledge—>attitude—>behavior causal sequence
is widely assumed to be correct.

Increasingly popular have been humanistic programs which variously seek to
change feelings, enhance self-esteem, clarify values, improve social skills, etc.,
typically through a variety of experiential activities (Seif, 1990, ch. 1). The logic
underlying this approach can be summarized with this syllogism:

Major Premise: Alcohol abuse is the result of a poorly developed self-concept.
Minor Premise: "Program X" will rectify deficiencies in self-concept.
Conclusion: Therefore, "Program X" will reduce alcohol abuse. (Goodstadt, 1986,
                   p. 353)

Even if, for example, poor self-concept were both a necessary and sufficient
cause of alcohol abuse (a highly questionable assumption) and even if programs

designed to improve self-concept were effective (another highly questionable assumption), removing the cause will not automatically eliminate the consequence (alcohol abuse) because the latter has many causes.

Program Evaluation

Belief in education as a major vehicle to reduce social problems receives widespread support in American society. But neither confidence, laudable goals, diligent effort, nor the commitment of vast sums of money is adequate to ensure success (Nathan, 1983, p. 459). Regardless of the objectives, the target groups, the content or instructional methods, it is important to evaluate carefully the impact of alcohol education programs on students. Only in that way can we develop a secure foundation on which to design or choose programs.

Unfortunately, the vast majority of drug education programs reported in the literature lack any evaluation. Those evaluations which are reported are often flawed by inadequacies of either research design and/or analysis. Thus, the literature provides little data for guidance in the development or modification of programs. Because some program components can be expected to be more effective with certain types of students or in certain settings, careful evaluation should make it possible to specify the optimal conditions for maximum effectiveness.

A leading alcohol educator has asserted that "We are throwing millions of dollars away on good faith efforts and programs that use *think* work. Little research is available on what actually works" (Gonzales, 1988, p. A35, emphasis in original) because program evaluation is rarely conducted.

Furthermore, it is not enough merely to demonstrate that a program is effective, or doing some good. "Efforts have to be made to assess how much good, to whom, why, and at what cost" (Grant, 1985, p. 311). Another educator observed that "It is often difficult to discontinue any program if it does not have the desired effect because time and money have typically been invested. Also there is often a feeling among presenters that 'at least we are trying to do something about the problem'" (Engs, 1977, p. 44; see also Goodstadt, 1986, p. 351). And "doing something" (almost *anything*) can protect administrators and school districts from law suits charging negligence (Baer et al., 1994, p. 83). On the other hand, increasing calls for accountability suggest the need to demonstrate successful educational efforts. More importantly, "All of the educating in the world concerning alcohol will be futile unless it is assured that the programs are effective" (Archibald, 1985, p. 27).

Those programs that are evaluated are often not evaluated properly. For example, "It is not sufficient to claim that any particular [alcohol education] campaign was a 'success' because a lot of people were aware of it, approved of it or though that it might be beneficial" (Bagnall and Plant, 1987, p. 420). Those evaluations that do examine possible changes in knowledge, attitudes, or behaviors often lack such basic essentials as control groups, not to mention randomization and other characteristics (some would say, essentials) of good experimental design.

SUMMARY

Prohibitionist sentiment has re-emerged with a modified agenda—alcohol consumption. Given the failure of prohibition, the reduction-of-consumption approach now more typically calls for a variety of measures designed to reduce the availability of alcohol and reduce its consumption. This approach views the substance of alcohol negatively and its unofficial motto is "less is better."

The positive experience with alcohol enjoyed by the American colonists, reinforced by the practice of Italians, Greeks, Jews and many others who immigrated to this country, provide the foundation of the sociocultural approach to alcohol. This approach views the problem as the abuse of alcohol, not alcohol itself. Therefore, attempts are made to eliminate alcohol abuse rather than alcohol when used in moderation.

Contemporary alcohol education has been heavily influenced by the abstinence legacy of Scientific Temperance Instruction. It has also been influenced by the dramatic rise in antidrug education, of which it has become a component.

In addition to the reduction-of-consumption versus responsible use debate, basic issues faced in developing an alcohol education include the objectives, the target group, the teaching personnel, and the content and methods. All too often the very important issue of program evaluation is ignored. The following chapter is entirely devoted to the important issue of evaluation.

NOTES

1. As Zimmer and Morgan (1992) point out, some writers have argued that prohibition had positive health consequences. Such writers (Aaron and Musto, 1981; Burnham, 1968; Gerstein, 1981; Kyvig, 1985; Moore, 1989) generally rely on data compiled by Warburton (1932) and Emerson (1932). However, Warbuton's data "clearly show that cirrhosis deaths began to decline as early as 1907, well before federal prohibition, and actually increased slightly during the latter years of prohibition," explain Zimmer and Morgan (1992, p. 1), who add "Emerson's cirrhosis data show a decline beginning in 1911, a more dramatic decline in the preprohibition years (1916–1919), and a slight increase during prohibition. Following prohibition's repeal, cirrhosis death rates were relatively stable until 1942 when they began to rise" (also see Miron and Zweibel, 1991). Furthermore, "The increase in the cirrhosis rate from 1922–1933 was also accompanied by similar increases in alcoholism deaths and alcohol psychosis" (Zimmer and Morgan, 1992, p. 1). They (p. 2) continue "We do not know if the increase in these adverse consequences was related to an increase in the number of drinkers or increased consumption of alcohol by a portion of those who drank illegally. What we do know is that consumption of distilled spirits increased during prohibition reversing a century long trend toward beer and wine (Hyman et al., 1980; Rorabaugh, 1979; Levine, 1984)."

2. Material in several of the following sections has been adapted from Hanson (1995, ch. 3).

3. Therefore, if reduction-of-consumption proponents wish to be technically correct, then drug-free schools with their oxygen-free environments would be an impossibility. Obviously they wish to be technically correct only when it suits their agenda. They sometimes call for drug-free environments while holding a cup of coffee in one hand and

a cigarette in the other.

4. One writer observed such strong and pervasive social pressure against social drinking that she declared hyperbolically that "Prohibition is in effect in New York, and the signs are everywhere" (Snowden, 1992, p. 131).

5. The Drug Free Schools and Communities Act was enacted in 1986 (P.L. 99–570). It was subsequently reenacted as Title V of the Elementary and Secondary Education Act (ESEA) of 1988 (P.L. 100–297). The Department of Education's Office of Elementary and Secondary Education administers Title V of ESEA, as amended by the Anti-Drug Abuse-Free Schools and Communities Act Amendment of 1989 and amendments to the Drug-Free Schools and Communities Act by the Crime Control Act of 1990 (U. S. Department of Education, 1993, p. 1).

6. In the opinion of one observer, "When programmes are established with the ostensible objective of changing attitudes, what is really meant is changing behavior. However, programmes designed to change behavior sound too harsh, drastic and politically dangerous: this is why they are eschewed" (Whitehead, 1979, p. 86). Perhaps the same is true of programs that state as their only objective that of increasing knowledge.

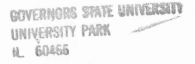

3

The Effectiveness
of Alcohol Education

Given the essential importance of outcomes assessment to the improvement of alcohol education, this chapter examines the effectiveness of such programs as reported over the past fifteen years. It focuses on in-school programs for the general student body in which changes in alcohol knowledge, attitudes or behaviors are assessed. The review is divided into one section on no-use programs and a second for those that are largely responsible-use in orientation. It finds that responsible-use programs are clearly superior to no-use programs, the latter being remarkably ineffective.

A report titled "Alcohol education can prevent alcohol problems: A summary of some *unique* finding" (Gonzales, 1982, emphasis added) conveys a great deal in its title alone. The fact that success in alcohol education is unique should be cause for deep concern, but it is typically unknown by the public and ignored by alcohol educators. Some alcohol and drug education has even found to be counter-productive, a fact leading to the suggestion that such education:

should be organized so that it does not exacerbate matters. Public money could easily be better spent in [the] future than it has in the past. This necessitates two main changes. First, the limitations and possible damages of certain types of alcohol and drug education need to be more widely understood. Many teachers, youth leaders, parents and policy makers simply do not appear to understand that alcohol and drug education might be counterproductive. Second, future activities, especially large scale public initiatives, must be carefully devised on the basis of available evidence. (Bagnall and Plant, 1987, p. 420)

This chapter examines the available evidence regarding the effectiveness of alcohol education as reported in materials published from 1979–1995. In addition to books and articles, a special effort was made to identify relevant doctoral dissertations, master's theses and diverse fugitive literature. It is limited to in-school programs for general students (rather than high risk students, medical students, developmentally disabled students, or other special category students) that empirically assess student outcomes in alcohol knowledge, attitudes, or behaviors. The educational levels encompassed in the search extended from kindergarten through graduate school. Not included were programs primarily or exclusively driver educational in nature or those that examined the perceptions of effectiveness.

The search included, but was not limited to, the following data bases: Alcohol Information for Clinicians and Educators, America: History and Life, Arts and Humanities Citation Index, Dissertation Abstracts Online, Education Index, Educational Resources Information Center (ERIC), GPO Monthly Catalog, Medline, PREVline, Public Affairs Information Service International, Psychological Abstracts, RLIN, Social Planning/Policy & Development Abstracts, Social Sciences Index, Social SciSearch, Sociological Abstracts, and WorldCat (the OCLC data base available through FirstSearch). WorldCat alone includes over 30,000,000 items. The computer-assisted components of the search were conducted in collaboration with an information specialist.

The chapter is divided into two sections. The first section presents programs that have a no-use orientation. The second section analyzes those that are largely responsible-use in orientation. It reveals that responsible-use programs are demonstrably superior to no-use programs.

NO-USE PROGRAMS ARE GENERALLY INEFFECTIVE

No-use programs are, with the sole exception of increasing alcohol knowledge, generally ineffective. Of the 10 studies examining only the impact of such programs on knowledge, seven found them to increase knowledge, one found no increase, and two found inconsistent or mixed results. However, no-use programs tend to be ineffective in changing attitudes and behaviors. For example, of the three investigations examining solely attitudes, only one found a positive impact. Of the 28 studies examining the impact of such programs solely on the very important variable of alcohol use, four (14%) found significant positive impact, two (7%) found the programs to be counterproductive, 13 (45%) found them to have no impact, and ten (34%) found mixed results.

Many studies examine the impact of no-use programs on some combination of knowledge, attitudes, or behaviors. Of the12 studies examining the impact of such programs on both knowledge and attitudes—but not on behaviors—two (17%) found significant impact on knowledge and attitudes, two found no impact, while eight (67%) found mixed (including counterproductive) effects. Of the eight investigations of knowledge and behavior (but not of attitudes), three (40%) found no influence from no-use programs, while 60% found only knowledge to be changed. In none of the eight studies was actual behavior changed. Of the six investigations of attitude and behavior (but not of knowledge), the results were even worse; four (67%) found no impact, one found only attitudes to be changed and one found negative (counterproductive) effects on both attitude and behavior. Again, in no case was there a positive impact on behavior. Finally, of the 23 studies of the impact of no-use programs on all three variables of knowledge, attitude, and behavior, only three (13%) found them to be successful with all three variables, whereas the remaining studies (87%) found either no impact or mixed impact.

Knowledge Increase is Only Success of No-Use Programs

While there is little reason to believe that knowledge is clearly or directly related to behavior, some studies have focused entirely on the cognitive dimension of alcohol education. Typically, investigations (70%) find that such education is associated with increases in knowledge about alcohol. For example, the effectiveness of an alcohol education curriculum in increasing knowledge among sixth, seventh, and eighth graders in Utah was assessed among 112 students in four classrooms (Gainer-Constine, 1984). Four other classrooms with 84 students comprised the control group. Pre- and post-tests were administered and revealed that exposure to the curriculum was associated with a significant increase in knowledge about alcohol.

Similarly, the effect of an educational program on the knowledge of adolescents regarding the effects of alcohol, smoking, and nutrition on pregnancy was examined by using two health education classes at a public high school (McGranor, 1982). One class served as the experimental group while the other was the control group. Twenty-one pairs of students in the two classes were matched on selected demographic variables and an investigator-developed knowledge inventory was used for the pre- and post-test. Significant increases in alcohol knowledge were found between the experimental pre- and post-tests.

A study of college students involved 440 male freshmen and sophomores living in four separate residence hall units at a large state university in Illinois who were assessed to determine the effectiveness of educational programming in increasing alcohol knowledge (Logan, 1980). Two of the residential units were randomly selected as experimental groups to receive intensive alcohol education programming while the two control groups received no such programming. Pre- and post-tests were used to assess changes in knowledge about alcohol, which encompassed the five specific areas of alcoholism, beverage equivalency, driving, medical classification, and physiological effects. The experimental units demonstrated significant increases in four of the five alcohol knowledge categories; there were no significant increases in the control units (Logan, 1980, p. 66).

The effects of a three week alcohol and drug education course on attitudes of ninth grade students in a small midwestern town were studied by Lignell and Davidhizar (1991). The 180 students in the required course completed both pre- and post-tests; there was no control group. Although no tests of significance were reported, the authors reported that "The mean attitude score for the group of students changed in the desired direction after education indicating negative feelings toward drugs and alcohol use and abuse, poly-drug use, dependency, social pressure and media pressure, and more positive feelings about legal restrictions and education" (Lignall and Davidhizar, 1991, p. 35).

The effectiveness of an alcohol education course given to high school students in the area of Padera, Italy, was evaluated by analyzing 2,166 completed and linked pre- and post-tests (Salvagnini et al., 1983). While no control group was used, analysis of test results indicated significant gains in nine of the ten knowledge questions.

Brooks (1992) tested the effects of lecture, cooperative learning, and independent learning methods on college students' alcohol knowledge. Ninety-three students at the University of Wyoming were randomly assigned to a lecture, cooperative learning, independent learning, or control condition for one semester. Pre- and post-tests revealed that all three experimental groups demonstrated significant increases in alcohol knowledge, with the lecture method producing the greatest gain.

Data on alcohol knowledge were collected from 665 eighth graders at five school districts in the Pacific Northwest whose pre- and post-tests were subsequently linked by a self-generated identification code. Knowledge about alcohol was measured by 12 information-oriented questions about the substance. Exposure to the program was associated with significant increases in alcohol knowledge; unfortunately, there was no control group to compare the observed increases (Weisheit et al., 1984).

However, not all investigators have found no-use alcohol education to increase knowledge. For example, an alcohol and drug education curriculum used with about 1,800 students in grades seven through nine was evaluated in 25 Nebraska junior high schools. Both experimental and control students completed pre- and post-tests. The results indicated that when the curriculum was taught by specially prepared (three day workshop) teachers, it significantly increased the alcohol knowledge of students aged 14 and 15, but not of those aged 12 and 13 (Newman et al., 1984).

The impact of Drug Abuse Resistance Education (DARE) on alcohol knowledge among elementary school children was examined in three school districts (Johnson, 1994). Two hundred eight students in the fifth and sixth grades were exposed to the 16 week curriculum while 44 served as controls. Pre- and post- tests revealed significant increases in knowledge among DARE students in two of the three districts.

A study at a private coeducational boarding school examined the impact of a six week alcohol education course on the alcohol knowledge of twelfth graders (Arndt, 1979). The twelve students were enrolled in a health education class and were pre- and post-tested; there was no control group. The results failed to indicated any increase in alcohol knowledge between the two tests.

Attitudes Resistant to No-Use Programs

Three studies have examined the impact of alcohol education on attitudes alone. Two (67%) found no change while one study reported a positive impact. One of the three studies was an experimental evaluation of Project PRIDE (Positive Results in Drug Education) that was conducted in Philadelphia by randomly assigned fifth through seventh graders to PRIDE and non-PRIDE conditions (LoSciuto and Ausetts, 1988). Project PRIDE attempts to increase students' self-awareness and life skills through small group counseling sessions and it also attempts to influence the "significant others" in the students' lives through training modules for parents and for teachers. Analyses of pre- and post-test results from 743 students revealed that while there was a significant increase in positive attitude toward beer, this increase was less pronounced among those who participated in the educational program. Unfortunately, data on alcohol use were not analyzed separately from those of other substances and cannot be interpreted (LoSciuto and Ausetts, 1988).

In another study, the attitudinal effects of the Beginning Alcohol and Addiction Basic Education Studies (BABES) curriculum was assessed among 68 eighth grade students in a Michigan junior high school. Forty-four eighth graders from a comparable school constituted the control group (Garcia-McDonnell, 1993). Results of the pre- and post-tests indicated no change in attitudes as a result of participation in the BABES program.

Finally, to determine the effect of a preventive alcohol education program of the attitudes of sixth grade students toward the consumption of alcohol, Bonilla (1993) studied 37 sixth graders at a middle school in rural South Carolina. The intervention group consisted of the 20 students in one classroom while the control group was composed of the 17 students in another classroom at the same school. There was no change in attitudes between pre- and post-testing.

Use of Alcohol Usually Unchanged by No-Use Programs

By far the most important test of educational effectiveness involves subsequent alcohol related behavior. Only four studies (14%) that examined solely behavior found no-use alcohol education to have an impact on actual use. One study was an assessment of a health curriculum for elementary school children that involved 600 students in two New York school districts who were pre-tested in kindergarten (Andrews and Hearne, 1984). The 284 students in experimental classrooms received an activity centered experential program. The 316 control group students received a standard teacher/textbook directed health education program. Post-testing data collected at the end of third grade indicated that self-reported drinking among the experimental group children was significantly less than that reported among the control group.

Another study focused on a social influence program. Social influence alcohol and drug programs are designed to teach social skills and to create a social environment less receptive to the use of alcohol and drugs. One such program, (the Midwestern Prevention Project) studied over 5,000 sixth and seventh graders in Kansas City, Missouri, and Kansas City, Kansas. Pre- and post-test results indicated a decreased proportion of experimental students reported using alcohol after the program (MacKinnon et al., 1991).

A third study was an assessment of seventh graders from two New York City schools who participated in a nine month study investigating the impact of an alcohol education program emphasizing decision-making, coping skills, social skills, and self-improvement (Botvin, 1984a). The two schools were randomly assigned to experimental and control conditions and students were given a pre-test, post-test, and six month follow-up test regarding drinking behaviors. Data from 167 students indicated that significantly more students in the experimental group reported less frequent drinking, less drinking per occasion, and less frequent intoxication than students in the control group.

The investigators stressed that:

The extent to which the preventive gains achieved over the course of this study can be sustained during the remainder of junior- and senior-high-school years is unclear. Our earlier research on cigarette smoking suggests that some form of ongoing intervention may be necessary to avoid a gradual erosion of the effects of this type of program. (Botvin et al., 1983)

Moreover, because only one school was assigned to the experimental and control condition, school and treatment effects are confounded, raising the possibility that these results may be at least partly the product of unmeasured school or teacher factors. Further research clearly needs to be conducted with longer term follow-up and a larger number of schools. (Botvin et al., 1984a, p. 552)

Finally, the Adolescent Alcohol Prevention Trial is an eight year project to examine the potential of a peer pressure resistance skills and of a "correction of erroneous perception about the prevalence and acceptability of alcohol use" approach to alcohol education (Hansen and Graham 1991, p. 415). Longitudinal tests of these two strategies are currently being conducted with four separate cohorts of students—two receive initial programming during the fifth grade and two receive it during the seventh grade. All students attend one of twelve participating schools in southern California. An analysis of seventh grade pre-test scores with eighth grade post-test scores has suggested that the refusal skills approach has had no impact on alcohol use, whereas the "correction of erroneous perceptions about the prevalence and acceptability of alcohol use" approach has slowed the onset of drinking, although alcohol consumption has increased steadily for all groups.

A number of behavioral studies have reported findings that can be described as mixed. For example, a study to assess the impact of DARE on fifth grade students was conducted in Long Beach, California (Becker and Agopian, 1992). Pre- and post-tests were administered to a total of approximately 3,000 students, about half of which were experimental and half were control. The investigators reported (p. 288, emphasis in original) that "DARE was *unable* to prevent a broad variety of substance use by students, e.g., the use of cigarettes, alcohol, and inhalants." More specifically, among the sample the DARE experimental group maintained beer and spirits consumption, while the control group increased its consumption of those beverages. On the other hand, wine consumption increased among both groups.

Another study was an alcohol use prevention study based on a social skills/peer pressure resistance approach that randomly assigned students in 49 schools to experimental and control groups (Dielman et al., 1992). Students were pre- and post-tested and tracked individually over time. All students were post-tested at the end of the first year of program implementation with follow-up testing at the end of the next two years. The researchers found that experimental students who had used alcohol unsupervised "showed a significantly greater reduction than their control in the rate of increase in susceptibility to peer pressure, alcohol use, and alcohol misuse. This difference was not found among students without prior unsupervised use of alcohol" (Dielman et al., 1992, p. 233).

All sixth, seventh and eighth grade students taking health education in three public middle schools in Georgia constituted the population for an alcohol education effectiveness study (Cleckler, 1991). During the week immediately preceding the treatment program and during the first week after conclusion of the program students were administered a test regarding the use of alcohol and other substances. Each student created a unique identification number for both answer sheets, that made it possible to connect pre- and post-tests. The investigator hypothesized four differences in alcohol use between experimental and control students. However, only one hypothesis was supported: significantly fewer experimental students reported that they became drunk or very high from drinking alcohol more often during the weeks between the pre-test and post-test administration than during the month prior to the pre-test.

The Akershus Project was an effort to test three approaches to alcohol and drug education in Akershus County, Norway (Lavik, 1986). One experimental group of students was given an informational program, a second received a values clarification approach, while a third was selected for a participation program:

The intention of this method is that pupils themselves were to be real participants in the exploring of the drug problem both in school and in their local environment. The teachers should act as supervisors guiding the pupils when they are interviewing their friends or gathering information from key persons. Finally, they should put forward proposals about actions which could combat the drug problem.
The basic idea is that only real participation and responsibility can influence behavior. (Lavik, 1986, p. 50)

Over 2,000 students (ages 15 and 16) participated in the experimental and control groups and were pre- and post-tested. Based on the results, the investigator observed:

All the pupils showed an increase in total alcohol consumption from pre-test (February) to post-test (May). The abstainers/light drinkers in the program groups showed a statistically significant reduction as regards this increase compared with the control group. This was most marked in the 8th grade, especially among the girls. (Lavik, 1986, p. 60)

McAlister and colleagues conducted a study in which, in one of two junior high schools, students (about 340) were given special training in resisting pressures toward alcohol, tobacco, or drug use. In the control school no such training was provided (McAlister et al., 1980). In post-tests and follow-up tests over a two year period it was found that there was a significantly higher incidence of control students who reported being high or drunk on alcohol during the previous day or week. However, there was no difference in the proportion of students who reported less frequent use of alcohol.

A cognitive/affective drug education program for high school students was assessed at a private religious school in a large midwestern city (Mitchell et al., 1984). Two hundred nine ninth grade students were experimental while 41 were controls. Data were collected on four test occasions: the pre-test, post-test, first follow-up, and second follow-up. The program was embedded in health, religion, and social studies classes. At the time of the second follow-up, only those students exposed to the program connected with religion classes reported any significant decrease in the use of any alcohol beverage, specifically liquor. There was no difference in the consumption of beer or wine.

Baer and colleagues (Baer et al., 1988) evaluated the effectiveness of two preventive programs on alcohol use among junior and senior high school students. One program focused on resistance to peer pressure, while the other stressed attitude change and decision making. The over 1,000 seventh graders and almost 1,500 tenth graders enrolled in these courses (along with control students), completed a pre-test. Seventh graders completed a two year follow-up while tenth graders completed a one year follow-up. The tenth grade one year follow-up data revealed that alcohol usage (last month, last year, and use per occasion) increased significantly among both experimental groups and the control group, although the relative increase was generally less for the intervention groups. The seventh grade two year follow-up failed to reveal any effect on any measure of usage for either educational program.

London and Duquette (1989) tested the effects of an alcohol education program based on Dennison's Activated Health Education (AHE) Model (Dennison, 1974, 1977). The model consists of an experential phase, followed by a cognitive phase and an affective phase to encourage students to take responsibility for their health regimens. Pre- and post-test data from a university alcohol education class based on AHE were compared to data from a traditional drug education (drugs and health) class, at the same university. Two alcohol related behavioral dependent variables were: (1) number of drinks consumed and (2) number of drinking problems. The time period for each variable was the seven day period immediately prior to each day the tests were administered. Neither course was associated with a significant reduction in number of drinks consumed but both were associated with a significant reduction in drinking problems. The authors considered the traditional drug education course (which included a total of only three hours and 45 minutes of instruction on alcohol) to be a control group. That brief instruction was lecture format and the authors asserted that:

Given the poor record of the type of instruction used in the Drugs and Health course in changing behavior, it would be difficult to argue convincingly that these reductions were indicative of effectiveness of both courses. More likely, the significant time of the semester effect can be explained better as a function of influences outside the classroom. For example, a natural student tendency to place a higher priority on studying toward the end of a semester than toward the beginning of a semester may result in a concomitant lowering of the priority of activities related to alcohol use. Alternatively, a maturation process occurring during a semester also might account for these reductions. (London and Duquette, 1989, pp. 32–33)

The Tobacco and Alcohol Prevention Project curriculum reflects an effort to combine successful prevention strategies into one educational package. Two school districts in the Los Angeles area participated in a test of its effectiveness (Hansen et al., 1987). In district A, two junior high schools were randomly selected to implement the curriculum. In district B, two schools—one treatment and one control—were selected. All students were pre-tested, then post-tested at the end of the course. Follow-up testing occurred one year, one and a half years, and two years after the course. There were no differences in drinking behavior between experimental and control students in district A. The investigators concluded that "The effects of the program on the prevalence of drinking in district B is not interpretable . . . [because] there is noncomparability with controls from the outset" (Hansen et al., 1987, p. 569). However, it appears that there was a gradual increase in drinking among treatment students and a slight decline among controls. Thus, the program appears to have been counterproductive.

The same curriculum was additionally tested for its impact on a total of 2,928 sixth and seventh grade students in Los Angeles county (Hansen et al., 1988a). Two cohorts of students were pre-tested and then tracked longitudinally. The first cohort was tested over a period of four years; the second was tested for three years. No effects of the program on alcohol use were detectable.

Hansen and his colleagues (1988b, p. 139) pointed out that "Affective education is based on the premise that many of the reasons for drug use initiation have to do with personal shortcomings (e.g., low self-esteem) and personal motivations (e.g., to feel better). Social influence programs, on the other hand, are quite clearly derived from a model that emphasizes external factors (e.g., role models and social pressures) as precipitators of drug use." They created an affective and a social influence program. Schools were then selected to receive one of the two semester long curricula or to serve as controls. There were 24 affective classrooms, 25 social classrooms, and 36 control classrooms, all at the seventh grade level. Students were pre-tested and then post-tested twelve and 24 months after the course was completed. The results indicated that the social influence program was generally effective in delaying the onset of alcohol consumption compared to the control condition. The prevalence of alcohol use was also lower in social influence classrooms than in control classrooms. On the other hand, the affective program had a negative impact "with all analyses at the first and second year follow-up measures indicating negative programmatic effects. By the final post-test, these effects were quite pronounced" (Hansen et al., 1988b, pp. 143–144). Thus, it was counterproductive.

The Midwestern Prevention Project was also studied by Pentz and colleagues (1989a). Pre-tests were administered to over 5,000 students in both experimental and control schools. Students were then assessed with post-tests and two annual follow-up tests. Reported alcohol use "last week" and "last month" was significantly lower among experimentals. While the proportion of both experimental and control students who reported consuming alcohol dramatically increased over time, that of experimentals did so at a lower rate (Pentz et al., 1989a). A lower proportion of experimental students using alcohol was also reported by MacKinnon and his colleagues (1991). However, analyses of test results from a subsample of over 1,600 of the students who were tracked individually over a three year period failed to identify any impact of the program on alcohol use (Johnson et al., 1990).

Other investigators assessing only behavior have found no-use alcohol education to be ineffective. For example, Ametrano (1992) examined the effects of a series of workshops designed to bring about a reduction of alcohol and other substance use by college freshmen. Students enrolled in four sections of a freshmen orientation course served as the experimental group while those enrolled in four other sections were the control group. A pre-test was administered to the 70 experimental and 66 control students. It was again administered immediately after the workshops were completed and two months later at the end of the semester. The resulting data revealed that the workshops had no effect on alcohol use.

Similarly, a study of 883 incoming freshmen students at three Massachusetts state colleges, representative of the population of the state as well as representative of all academic majors, found no significant relationships between the number of alcohol education courses in which the respondents were involved in kindergarten through twelfth grade and their alcohol related behavior (Dunn, 1981). Additionally, there was no significant relationship between the methods used to teach alcohol education courses in kindergarten through twelfth grade and three of four indices used to measure alcohol related behavior.

Seventh grade students in three inner city parochial schools participated in a study comparing a traditional program with an assertiveness drug prevention program (Dupont & Jason, 1984). Pre-test, post-test and six month follow-up test results revealed no significant change in alcohol consumption over time for the traditional, assertiveness, or control group.

In an effort to examine the effectiveness of prevention programs mandated by the Drug-free Schools and Community Act of 1989, Irwin (1994) conducted pre- and post-tests at two Catholic universities using the CORE Alcohol and Drug Survey self-report questionnaire (Presley et al., 1990), supplemented by additional items. No relationship was found between knowledge of alcohol policy programs on campus and alcohol consumption. A category measure termed "awareness' was then constructed combining knowledge of such programs or policies and a student self-report that prevention programs *have* caused the respondent to be less favorable toward and less likely to use alcohol and drugs. Perhaps this category should more accurately be described as being both aware and affected. Only about 18 percent of the student body of either institution were aware and affected. However, being aware and affected was significantly associated with quantity and frequency of drinking. Thus, students who report that they are less favorable toward and less likely to use alcohol are less likely to drink frequently or heavily.

While the study found a relationship between attitude and behavior, it did not demonstrate that alcohol education or policies affect drinking behaviors.

Another doctoral research project attempted to evaluate the impact of a series of alcohol education programs by comparing matched pairs in treatment and control groups (Zeller, 1985). Comparison of pre- and post-test results failed to reveal an impact of such programs on student drinking behaviors.

Zuelke (1993) examined the nature and prevalence of alcohol use among college seniors to determine if a correlation exists between those variables and exposure to alcohol and drug education courses by conducting a secondary analysis of data collected by the Monitoring the Future survey of high school students throughout the United States (Institute for Social Research, 1986). After controlling for gender and race, Zuelke (p. 64) concluded that "whether or not one received drug education did not affect alcohol consumption" and that "drug education programs neither promoted nor deterred alcohol consumption."

Four alcohol education programs having a social skills and self-concept focus were assessed for effectiveness by Bonaguro and colleagues (1988). Fifth through eighth graders in the participating rural Ohio schools completed pre- and post-tests. There was no program impact on alcohol (or other substance) use.

Because of a number of methodological flaws in DeJong's (1987) evaluation of Project DARE's effectiveness, Ringwalt and colleagues (1991) conducted a more rigorous test of outcomes. Fifth and sixth grade students from 20 schools in North Carolina participated in the study; ten (with 685 students) were randomly assigned to receive DARE program while ten (with 585 pupils) were designated control schools. Confidential pre- and post-tests were assigned unique identification numbers so that students' responses on the two tests could be linked. Analysis of the results indicated that DARE had no effect on student use of alcohol.

A study of seventh grade students at six intermediate schools who had participated in the DARE program as fifth graders was conducted in Honolulu (Hawaii State Department of Education, 1989). There were no significant differences in alcohol use between DARE and non-DARE students as determined by a post-test.

A study of 1,931 third and fourth graders from 20 Aukland, New Zealand, public high schools investigated the impact of a drug education program (Casswell, 1982). The results of pre- and post-testing indicated no significant impact of the program on the frequency of drinking or of intoxication.

Gersick and colleagues (1988) evaluated the effectiveness of a program based on interpersonal skill enhancement and decision-making among sixth graders. Six hundred ninety-eight experimental and 674 control students completed post-tests; no pre-tests were used. There were no significant differences between programs and control students on mean use levels of alcohol (or other substances). However, "controls demonstrated greater nonuse and lower experimental use than Program students" (Gersick et al., 1988, p. 64). Thus, the program appears to have been counterproductive.

Knowledge and Attitudes Generally Unaffected by No-Use Programs

Investigators often assess both alcohol knowledge and attitudes (but not behavior) as independent variables. However only two (17%) of these studies have found a positive effect of no-use alcohol education on both knowledge and attitudes. One such study sought to determine if a four month alcohol education program with a heavy emphasis on developing positive self-esteem could increase alcohol knowledge, attitudes and "behavior" among 84 fifth grade students who were pre- and post-tested with a ten item questionnaire (Miller, 1988). There was no control group. While none of the items addressed actual behavior; some examined hypothetical behavioral intentions that might be considered proxies for attitudes. For example "If your parents told you it was okay, would you use alcohol?" Significant change was found in all items. In the pre-test, 41.7 percent of students said they would consume alcohol with parental approval; only 1.2 percent of students gave the same response in the post-test. It would appear that the program was successful in increasing "knowledge" that they could die from using alcohol and that they cannot legally drink alcohol. Students appear to have been taught incorrectly that they cannot legally drink, given their ability to do so legally for religious purposes, or in their homes under parental supervision or in medications. The program was thus apparently successful in increasing "knowledge" and in changing attitudes.

The second study examined the impact of a program called "Here's Looking at You, 2000" ("Here's Looking at You" and "Here's Looking at You, Two," discussed later, are earlier versions of this program) on the knowledge and attitudes of elementary school students. The program was presented to a sixth grade class in a private school with another sixth grade class in the same school serving as a control (Chard-Yaron, 1992). Pre- and post-test results indicated that the program was successful in conveying the alcohol information and attitude components of the curriculum.

None of the other studies have found a positive effect of alcohol education on both knowledge and attitudes. For example, students in eighth grade classes who had been given a health education unit on alcohol were compared with eighth grade students who had not received such instruction in order to examine the impact of the unit on students' knowledge and attitudes regarding alcohol (Foerster, 1985). The experimental group of 117 students received the alcohol unit of study presented by their classroom teacher within a ten day period after the pre-test; the control group of 55 received a general health unit of study. At the end of the alcohol educational unit time period, all subjects were given the post-tests. While the knowledge post-test scores were significantly higher for the experimental group, the attitude post-test scores were not significantly different for the two groups.

A study to implement and rigorously evaluate a comprehensive alcohol education curriculum in grades four, five and six was conducted with 832 students in 36 classes in six school districts in Utah (Terry, 1982). Teachers participated in a three day alcohol education workshop and agreed to teach the curriculum during a three week period; they were then randomly assigned so that half were experimental and half were control at each grade level. Significant differences in alcohol knowledge favored the experimental groups at all grade levels. However, no overall changes in attitude occurred between pre- and post-testing and no significant differences existed between experimental and control groups.

Botvin's (1981) life skills training curriculum was evaluated with sixth graders by Kreutter and her colleagues (1991). One hundred fifty-two students from one school in Connecticut constituted the experimental group while 64 students from three other schools made up the control group. Pre- and post-tests, including investigator developed alcohol and drug knowledge and attitude scales, were administered to all subjects. The results indicated a significant increase in alcohol and drug knowledge among the experimental students; no results regarding attitudes were reported and are, therefore, presumably negative.

Klee (1982) examined the effectiveness of an alcohol and drug education program that emphasized values clarification, decision-making communication and interpersonal relationships. Approximately 500 adolescents (about 50 from each school) from study halls voluntarily participated in twelve one hour sessions. About 350 students (about 35 from each school) served as controls. All were pre- and post-tested. Results indicated that program participants significantly increased their knowledge of alcohol, but there were no significant changes in attitudes.

Two fraternity houses at a large New England state university participated in a study to examine the effects of a minimal cognitive intervention on alcohol related knowledge and attitudes of fraternity members (Bowling, 1991). A total of 48 members from both fraternity houses were administered a pre-test measure of alcohol related knowledge and attitudes and an alcohol use assessment packet. All tests were number coded and seven days later individual results were distributed to the subjects. Each subject received a two page summary of his alcohol use that presented specific assessment results, interpretations of results, individual risk factors, and relevant alcohol information (the concept of alcohol equivalency, the metabolic process of alcohol, etc.). Three days after subjects received assessment results, they were administered the post-test measure of knowledge and attitudes. Post-test data were obtained from 45 of the original 48 subjects and revealed a significant increase in alcohol knowledge. However, there was no change in attitudes.

Other studies were even less successful. For example, an alcohol education program was recently designed for pledges of Greek organizations at a large state university in the midwest (Trefethen, 1993). To determine its effects on student knowledge and attitudes, pre-, post-, and four week follow-up tests were administered to pledges, who were required to participate in the program. Post-test knowledge scores for males were significantly higher than either pre-test or follow-up scores. For females, knowledge scores on the post-test and follow-up test were significantly higher than the pre-test scores. Thus, males did not retain alcohol knowledge like the female subjects. However, the overall program had little impact on participants' attitudes about alcohol.

Similarly, a study of 797 fifth graders examined the effectiveness of the School Health Curriculum among elementary school children (Watts, 1982). The sample attended a public school in Richmond, Virginia and was predominantly black, urban, poor, and below the average age of onset of smoking and drinking. The experimental group of 464 students was exposed to the fifth grade unit of the School Health Curriculum for ten weeks while the control group of 333 received the regular health education classes. Results revealed that alcohol related knowledge increased significantly for students in the *control* group but *not* in the experimental group. More significantly, there were no differences between the two groups in their intentions to drink alcohol (conceptualized as attitudes). It might be noted that an experimental subgroup had received an additional decision implementation training module. In most instances students in this module actually lost ground, although their average change rates were not significantly different from those in the regular experimental group.

Five Omaha area Catholic High schools developed a cooperative program for a comprehensive alcohol education and counseling program to be implemented one day per week at each of the schools. Pre- and post-testing was conducted for alcohol knowledge and attitudes. There was no significance between experimental and control groups in either alcohol knowledge or attitudes (Burch, 1980).

Seventh grade students in two school systems in rural North Carolina were subjects in a program to reduce alcohol and tobacco use. The North Carolina Health Education Risk Reduction program was designed to prevent the onset of alcohol and tobacco use among adolescents as well as to reduce the prevalence of these behaviors when already existing among students (Dignan et al., 1985). Teaching methods included lectures, demonstrations, role playing, film, exercises, reading, homework and examinations. The approximately 2,300 students received pre- and post-tests to assess knowledge and attitudes. There were no control groups. Alcohol knowledge increased significantly in both school systems. Alcohol attitudes changed significantly in only one system, and that change was in a negative direction. Thus, the program appears to have been, on balance, counterproductive.

All 37 sixth graders in a small Iowa elementary school participated in an alcohol education program emphasizing decision-making and parental involvement and support. There was no control group. Analysis of pre- and post-testing revealed no significant differences over time in either alcohol attitudes or behaviors (Schach, 1990).

Knowledge and Behavior Changed Little by No-Use Programs

As a group, studies examining the impact of alcohol education on knowledge and behavior (but not on attitudes) report very discouraging findings. Of eight studies, three (40%) found no impact on either knowledge or behavior. The rest found change only in knowledge. In none of the studies was behavior changed.

The purpose of Pamela Collins' (1980) study was to examine the short-term and long-term effects of a peer education program on education emphasizing decision making on seventh graders' knowledge and involvement with alcohol. All subjects received instruction through the regular health education unit on alcohol taught by a classroom teacher. Subsequently, the experimental group received additional instruction through the Allied Youth Peer Education Program taught by high school peer instructors. It was found that subjects who received instruction through the Peer Education Program received higher mean scores on knowledge of alcohol information than did subjects who simply received instruction through the regular health education unit. However, there were no significantly different patterns of use or abuse of alcohol between the experimental and the control groups.

A five year demonstration alcohol education project at an eastern state university used methods that included "community development, mass media, and such intensive approaches as workshops, courses, and guest lectures" (Duston, et al., 1981, p. 272). A survey of a sample of the total student body was taken annually supplemented by a survey of students completing a three credit alcohol education course. Data from the alcohol course indicated that they significantly increased their knowledge about alcohol. However, successive surveys of the student body failed to reveal any positive changes in drinking behaviors or problems resulting from drinking.

One hundred eighty-nine students in the sixth grade who attended eight elementary schools in Salt Lake City participated in an alcohol and drug education research project. The curriculum "presented information on the immediate, negative effects of nicotine, alcohol, and marijuana and taught skills in responsible decision-making and resisting social persuasion" (Durrant, 1986, p. iv). Four classes were randomly assigned to the experimental group and the four remaining classes became the control group. All participants completed a pre- and post-test on knowledge and behavior. The results indicated that the treatment group, compared to the control group, experienced a significant gain in knowledge of the immediate negative effects of alcohol and drug use but no difference in the use of alcohol, which did not change.

Newman and his colleagues (1992, p. 55) correctly pointed out that "When the goals of an education program are to inform *and* to change behavior, it is important to evaluate the success of both." With this in mind they evaluated a ninth grade alcohol education program developed on the basis of problem behavior therapy, social cognitive theory, and role theory. Its goals were to increase knowledge and to reduce drinking, drinking and driving, and riding with a drinking driver. The program was taught to half of the 84 ninth grade classes in all nine junior high schools in Nebraska city while the other half served as controls. Students' knowledge and behaviors were assessed before, immediately after, and one year after completion of the two year program. The investigators (Newman et al., 1992) found significant increases in knowledge associated with those who took the course. However, both experimental and control students significantly increased their consumption of alcohol, their frequency of consumption, and "having more to drink at the last party they attended." While both groups reported riding a greater number of times with a drinking driver, the increase in the experimental group was significantly less than that of the control group. This differential persisted to the follow-up test.

In a study of educational effectiveness, 56 junior high schools in New York State were randomly assigned to receive (a) the prevention program with formal teacher training and feedback regarding this implementation of the curriculum, (b) the prevention program with videotaped teacher training and no feedback, or (c) no program (Botvin et al., 1990). The Life Skills Training Program was the educational program implemented:

It teaches students cognitive-behavioral skills for building self-esteem, resisting advertising pressure, managing anxiety, communicating effectively, developing personal relationships, and asserting one's rights. These skills are taught using a combination of teaching techniques including demonstration, behavioral rehearsal, feedback and reinforcement, and behavioral "homework" assignments for out-of-class practice. (Botvin et al., 1990, p. 439)

Students in the program additionally received annual booster courses after the first course. All of the 4,466 students in the study received a pre- and post-test with one year, two year, and three year follow-up tests. Results indicated that students in the experimental conditions had significantly more alcohol knowledge than did those in the control group. Although they reported drinking as frequently and as much as control students, experimental students reported less frequent intoxication.

A Swedish study (Bremberg and Arborelius, 1994) examined the impact of an alcohol education program regularly taught to ninth graders in the public schools of Linkoping (population 120,000). Teachers recruited 65 volunteer students to participate in the study and matched other students to constitute a control group. Pre-tests, post-tests and follow-up tests were connected with identification codes. The results revealed no significant difference between the experimental and control groups on either alcohol knowledge or consumption. The investigators (Bremberg and Arborelius, 1994, p. 118) noted in particular the lack of impact on behavior and observed that: "The same is true of most other approaches to school based alcohol prevention aiming at mid adolescents. From this perspective, it is somewhat bewildering that alcohol education is at all continued in schools."

Project ALERT is a social-influence program for seventh and eighth grades that attempts to curb the use of alcohol, cigarettes, and marijuana that was subjected to a methodologically sophisticated test of effectiveness (Ellickson & Bell, 1990; Ellickson et al., 1993). Thirty highly diverse schools were randomly selected from California and Oregon. Students completed questionnaires about alcohol and drug attitudes and behaviors four times during grades seven and eight. Testing was conducted before and after the educational program as well as before and after eighth grade booster lessons. The results suggested no program success in changing alcohol knowledge or in expectancies regarding future use of alcohol. The program "yielded modest inroads against drinking in grade 7, but those gains eroded within 12 months" and "the program had no impact on cigarette and alcohol expectations [regarding future use] during year 2" (Ellickson et al., 1993, pp. 228 and 234). The researchers (Ellickson et al., 1993, pp. 239–240) observed that:

the program's more limited impact on alcohol use and beliefs suggests that this kind of curriculum will be most effective when societal mores and attitudes reinforce the message. Program activities aimed at making drinking less socially acceptable were clearly contradicted by the students' own experience: before Project ALERT began, almost three fourths of the students had tried alcohol and 74% reported that at least one parent or sibling drinks. Even after exposure to project ALERT, students in the treatment schools believed that nearly half of their peers were current drinkers—and that belief reflected reality. We might have observed additional program effects on alcohol-related beliefs had we obtained specific measures about the social consequences of drinking. But if such effects did, in fact, occur, they clearly were not enough to change behavior in the face of the entrenched perception that drinking is the norm.

Our research suggests that equipping young people with skills to resist pro-drinking pressure is not the problem: the techniques they learn for resisting cigarettes or marijuana apply to alcohol as well. What they need, and appear to lack, is the support for using those skills—from other peers, family members, and the broader community,. Additional school, community, and media efforts to deglamorize alcohol use and to promote drug-free activities for teenagers would likely enhance the program's effectiveness.

A follow-up study conducted when students reached the ninth grade revealed no change in the program's ineffectiveness regarding alcohol knowledge or behavior (Bell et al., 1993).

Attitudes and Behaviors Resistant to No-Use Programs

Six studies have examined the impact of alcohol education on attitudes and behavior (but not knowledge). Four (67%) found no impact on either attitudes or behaviors, one found a change only in attitude, while one found a negative (counterproductive) change in both attitude and behavior. Thus, in no case was there a positive impact on actual behavior.

One study was conducted to determine the effects on students' attitudes and behavior of contracted abstinence—signing a pledge not to drink any alcohol for a certain period of time—and a course on alcoholism. Participants were undergraduate psychology students enrolled in either a five week summer session class on psychosocial aspects of alcoholism ("class") or a regular semester course in introductory psychology ("non-class"). A total of 92 students divided into four conditions (class/abstinence, class/no abstinence, no class/abstinence, and no class/no abstinence). Pre- and post-test measures of attitudes toward alcohol use as well as self-reported drinking behavior (using an instrument in which students kept a daily record of the amount and type of beverage drunk, the setting and social situation where drinking occurred, the number of drinks refused, and the cost of the day's drinking) were used. The resulting data led the researchers to conclude that:

contracted abstinence has little systematic effect on attitude change regarding alcohol use in college students. While both the alcohol class and abstinence experience have some potency in modifying college students' self-reported drinking behavior, it appears that the contracted abstinence has an impact only when it is incorporated in an alcohol class. (Blum et al., 1980, p. 76)

In another study, 120 students in the sixth grade were used in an analysis of the effectiveness of the Meeks-Heit Drug and Alcohol Education Curriculum (Meeks and Heit, 1986). This kindergarten through twelfth grade health curriculum has three chapters in the drug unit at the sixth grade level: (1) Some Facts about Drugs, (2) Alcohol and Tobacco, and (3) Making Responsible Choices. In this study, the curriculum was augmented with refusal skill training and adaptive coping strategies. The 60 experimental students were in one school district while the 60 control students were in another. All students were pre- and post-tested. There were no significant differences between the experimental and control groups in alcohol attitudes on completion of the educational program. The experimental groups experienced no significant difference in alcohol behaviors between the pre- to post-tests while the control groups showed a significant difference in behavior. The author explained that "the shift was in a negative direction. The pre-test mean scores for behavior were high indicating anti-alcohol behaviors, therefore a stable mean score in the experimental group post-test indicated negative alcohol behaviors were not developing as was seen in the control group," and concluded that "the drug program may have held the positive alcohol behavior stable in the experimental group" (Cooper, 1989, pp. 60–61).

The effects of a drug and alcohol education program implemented at a state university in Minnesota were examined over a two-year span using self-reported alcohol/drug use attitudes and behaviors (Jorgensen, 1990). Survey comparisons before and after implementation of the educational program found no significant change in attitudes and behaviors over the two year period.

A study of 232 residence hall students at a Minnesota state university compared the attitudes and behaviors of those who voluntarily participated in an alcohol education program in the hall with those who chose not to participate (Reall, 1989). No control group or pre-testing was used in this study, which found no significant differences in alcohol attitudes or behaviors between the participating and non-participating students.

To assess the impact of DARE on attitudes toward drugs and self-reported substance use among sixth graders, 23 schools were randomly selected to receive the DARE curriculum while eight were randomly designated as controls (Clayton et al., 1991). All students completed a pre- and post-test, the results of which revealed an impact of DARE in increasing anti-drug attitudes. Importantly, however, there were no differences between DARE and non-DARE students in reported use of alcohol.

To examine the impact of an cognitive/affective drug education program on alcohol beliefs and behaviors, Sarvela and McClendon (1987) studied 265 rural sixth graders. All sixth grade students in one school served as the experimental subjects while all those in a neighboring school were the controls. Analysis of pre- and post-test results indicated a significant increase in favorable attitude toward alcohol consumption and, more importantly, a significant increase in frequency of alcohol consumption among those who took the course.

Knowledge, Attitudes, Behaviors Little Affected by No-Use Programs

Many studies have examined the effectiveness of no-use alcohol education on the three dependent variables of alcohol knowledge, attitudes, and behaviors. However, only three investigations (14%) have found an effect on all three variables. In one such study, Gliksman and his colleagues (1983) evaluated the effectiveness of the satirical theatrical performance *Booze* on ninth and tenth grade students' alcohol knowledge, attitudes, and behavior. *Booze* consists of five skits largely focusing on alcohol problems. All students received a pre-test and the same instrument as a post-test about one week after the intervention. It measures a students' alcohol knowledge, attitudes, and behavior. The authors describe their procedure:

In addition to comparing those students receiving the performance to a control group, the students were compared to a group of students who had been given similar information via the traditional didactic manner, and with a group of students who received both the performance and the traditional method. Thus, the impact of the theatrical performance could be evaluated against a group receiving no alcohol education, a group receiving traditional education, and a group receiving both approaches (in order to determine whether or not the effects of such an approach are additive).

It was hypothesized that the theatrical program would have a positive impact (when compared to the control group) on these students' knowledge, attitudes, motivation, and behaviors with respect to alcohol. That is, they would become more knowledgeable, develop less positive attitudes towards alcohol, be less motivated to use alcohol, and reduce their consumption. However, comparisons with the other experimental groups were not subject to a prior hypothesis because of the novel nature of the intervention and comparisons. (Gliskman et al., 1983, p. 231)

Seven hundred sixteen students completed both the pre- and post-test. The results suggested that, at least in the short run, the one hour live theatrical performance was generally as effective in influencing knowledge, attitudes, and behaviors. The results were the same for the four-hour formal presentation.

Caleekal-John and Pletsch (1984) investigated the effects of a two week alcohol education unit on university students' alcohol knowledge, attitudes, and behaviors. No control group was used in this study. The 17 drinkers in the course completed pre- and post-tests and a one month follow-up test. The resulting data indicated that the education unit significantly increased alcohol knowledge and "responsible" (i.e., negative or anti-alcohol) attitudes. The follow-up test revealed that those increases persisted as well as a reduced incidence of negative consequences of alcohol use.

A unique teaching approach, Teams-Games-Tournaments (TGT), is based on a behavioral group work perspective and utilizes peer support and emphasizes group, rather than individual, achievement (Wodarski, 1981; Wodarski, 1987, see pp. 125–129 for a succinct description of the approach). It was assessed using five Georgia school systems in which 570 students received instruction using the TGT method, 384 received traditional instruction, and 411 received no instruction. Comparison of pre- and post-test results indicated that the experimental classes had significant increases in alcohol knowledge compared to the other classes. Experimental classes exhibited a significantly greater positive attitude change than did the other classes. They also significantly decreased their consumption of alcohol. A follow-up indicated that these changes persisted for at least two years (Wodarski, 1986–1987; 1987; Wodarski and Bordnick, 1994).

A program emphasizing alcohol refusal skills was examined among all eighth grade students in selected schools in Australia (N=828), Chile (N=195), and Norway (N=1306) as well as all ninth graders (N=207) in selected Swaziland schools (Perry, 1989). Schools within each country were randomly assigned to peer-led, teacher-led, or control conditions. Analysis of pre- and post-test results revealed that "Overall, the peer-led program demonstrated significantly lower alcohol use scores than the teacher-led and control conditions for both non-drinkers ($p<0.003$) and drinkers ($p<0.04$)" (Perry, 1989, p. 58). Although no data were presented, it was reported that students in the peer-led condition also gained more knowledge and acquired better attitudes than did others.

Most studies examining the impact of no-use alcohol education on knowledge, attitudes, and behaviors have found mixed results. Given the relative ease in increasing knowledge, it is not surprising that the majority of such investigations found changes in knowledge but not in attitudes or behaviors. An example is Collins' (1990) study of the effects on alcohol knowledge, attitudes, and behaviors of an alcohol education presentation and of the presentation including a public service announcement component (Collins, 1990; Collins and Cellucci, 1991). The presentations were made over a three day period to tenth and eleventh grade students in rural South Carolina. Fifty-two students were assigned to either of two treatment groups or a control group. Both treatment groups received the same educational presentation but one also received the public service announcements. All students received a pre-test, a post-test, and a one month follow-up test. Although all groups exhibited significantly increased knowledge scores from pre- to post-tests, only the experimental groups maintained this increase one month later. There were no significant differences in either alcohol attitudes or behaviors associated with either educational program.

One hundred and fifty-five ninth grade students participated in a study investigating student tendency to comply with peers in various risky alcohol and driving situations. Experimental students received a one week preventive alcohol education treatment:

The intervention for the study consisted of film, question/answer, role playing and slide show presentation. The film addressed the physiological effects of alcohol on bodily performance. The question/answer session followed the film and was designed to reinforce the major content of the film. The role play exercise allowed students to act out alcohol related situations in which they were subjected to adult, sibling and peer pressure to comply in risky drinking and driving episodes. The slide show presentation subsequently reviewed the major ideas explored in each of the three prior treatments. During the slide show students were shown slides depicting various drinking and driving concepts (i.e., one showed a person amidst numerous empty beer cans drinking coffee). After each slide students were asked to explain the accompanying concept (i.e., only time not coffee helps return sobriety).

Each of the treatments lasted approximately one hour per day for one week. Participating teachers were trained to implement the program in a series of workshops conducted by the author.

All four of the study treatments were designed to emphasize two central themes to students: (1) Alcohol impairs bodily performance and nothing except the passage of time will help speed the sobering-up process and, (2) no person must conform or comply with pressure to partake in risky behavior. (Duryea, 1985, p. 45)

Results indicated that the experimental students experienced significantly greater gains in knowledge but not in attitudes or behaviors (Duryea, 1983; 1985).

At a six month follow-up, the extent to which the initial program outcomes persisted among students in the experimental groups was assessed. There were seven dependent measures in his study: (1) students' skill in refuting persuasive alcohol related arguments, (2) frequency of drinking alcohol, (3) frequency of riding with drinking drivers, (4) tendency to comply in risky alcohol-related situations with peers, (5) frequency of refusing to ride with drinking drivers, (6) frequency of refusing a drink of alcohol, and (7) frequency of accepting a drink of alcohol. The last three dependent variables—refusing a drink, accepting a drink, and refusing to ride—were not included in the original study (Egwaoje, 1982, p. 5). The six month follow-up revealed that experimental students continued to avoid riding with drinking drivers, and continued to report the tendency to avoid risky alcohol related situations. However, there were no significant differences in terms of refusing to ride with drinking drivers, in refusing a drink of alcohol, or in accepting a drink of alcohol (Egwaoje, 1982; Duryea et al., 1984).

At a three year follow-up, another assessment of the original students (then in the eleventh grade) was conducted. The investigators examined frequency of riding with a drinking driver, frequency of drinking alcohol, frequency of drinking too much alcohol, and responses to two alcohol knowledge items (Duryea and Okwumabua, 1988). There was only one significant difference on these five items between experimental and control students, and that was in the unintended direction: control students reported less frequently drinking to excess than did those who had been in the alcohol education program. Thus over time, it appears to have been counterproductive.

To determine which of three methods of alcohol education is most likely to increase alcohol knowledge, modify attitudes, and change drinking behavior, students at a midwestern post-secondary two year vocational-technical institution were studied (McManus, 1980). One treatment group was self-selected while another was volunteered by a general education course instructor as was the control group. The first treatment group was exposed to the film *Booze and Yous*. The second treatment group was exposed to the same film and also participated in values clarification discussion exercises. The anonymous self-report inventory was administered as a pre-test to all groups, as a post-test to the experimental groups at the completion of their alcohol education program, and as an eight week post-test to all groups. Immediately following participation in alcohol education, significant increases in alcohol knowledge were found for both experimental groups but not for the control group. The group participating in values clarification discussion exercises demonstrated the greater increase in knowledge. No differences in attitudes or behaviors were found. Data collected eight weeks later revealed that both the control groups retained alcohol knowledge, with retention being greater for the values clarification group.

Robinson and her colleagues (1993) compared five week psychoeducational classes on substance abuse with control classes to determine if the psycho-educational classes would influence the substance use knowledge, attitudes, and behaviors of college students. The investigators described the experimental treatment:

The primary focus of these five-week modules was adolescent substance abuse, with lectures emphasizing family, school, and personal variables influencing at risk behaviors, the historical development of America's drug problem, the psychophysiological impact of drugs, other drug information such as signs, symptoms and consequences of specific drug use, and prevention and intervention programs. Substances which were discussed included tobacco, alcohol, marijuana, cocaine, inhalants, stimulants, depressants, and hallucinogens.

Students were given textbook readings and handouts to prepare for each class period, and during the majority of class time, the instructor presented information to enhance the readings. Because of the nature of the topics being covered and the age of the students (most in late adolescence themselves), class discussions which allowed students not only to clarify the meaning and implications of the presented material but for them to ask "what if" questions were encouraged. (Robinson et al., 1993, p. 125)

Fifty of 54 experimental and 49 of 53 control subjects completed both pre- and post-tests. Results indicated that while the experimental classes significantly increased knowledge about substances, they failed to impact either attitudes or behaviors.

An experimental examination of three approaches to alcohol education compared a cognitive program, a decision-making program, and a values clarification program (Goodstadt and Sheppard, 1983). Each of the programs consisted of ten lessons taught during consecutive daily health classes by staff from the Addiction Research Foundation of Toronto, Ontario. A total of 332 students participated in the three experimental programs; an additional 208 students served as controls. Knowledge, attitudes, and behaviors were assessed by means of pre-tests, post-tests and a six month follow-up test. The cognitive program increased levels of alcohol knowledge significantly more than did the other programs, but no significant differences between the programs was found in attitude change and in reported alcohol use.

Elwood (1991) analyzed the impact of the DARE curriculum on sixth grade students' alcohol knowledge, attitudes, and behaviors. Eighty-two students in a midwestern school district were studied (Elwood, 1991); 44 experimental subjects attended one elementary school while 38 control group subjects attended another. An alcohol use questionnaire was used as both the pre- and post-test. Results indicated a significant difference between the experimental and control group means in alcohol knowledge and attitudes. The data did not indicate a significant difference between the groups in alcohol behavior.

An alcohol and drug education program based on the philosophy that both peers and teachers have a significant influence on students' attitudes and behaviors regarding alcohol and drugs, was designed and implemented in a ninth and tenth grade public school in a southwestern state (Argentos, 1991). The program was given to the entire student body of 743 students, half were both pre- and post-tested. A control group of 70 students of similar demographics was randomly selected from another school in the same community. The educational program included extensive teacher training, heavy involvement of student leaders, and six hours of prevention curricula for five days. Program activities included:

presentation of factual information, open-ended discussion groups, video tapes, speakers, a poster campaign, involvement with newspaper and television media, a door-decorating contest, an anti-drug t-shirt wearing contest, coke and pizza parties, and a school-wide rally. All of these activities were designed to reflect a philosophy of drug prevention which highlights a "marketing approach" to change attitudes through social influence. In all, students participated in thirty-six hours of drug-preventive "inoculation." A significant aspect of the "marketing approach" included red t-shirts with an anti-drug slogan provided by local merchants. Students were able to obtain the shirts by paying two dollars and signing a pledge to remain drug free for the program duration. (Argentos, 1991, p. 23)

The day after this intensive no-use program ended, students were post-tested, staff and administration received a "retrospective pretest and post- test" to determine their observations regarding changes in student attitudes, and a short "retrospective pretest/post-test" was given to a convenience sample of parents. Six months after the educational program, 140 students were randomly selected for testing to determine if program effects remained. At the end of the program, those exposed to it reported significantly higher levels of knowledge about popular myths concerning alcohol and significantly more negative attitudes toward alcohol. However, there were no significant differences between experimental and control groups in reported behaviors, such as the use of alcohol or riding with an impaired driver. Interestingly, the parental and staff/administration surveys demonstrated the perception of program success. Six months later, following and during booster components of the program, alcohol knowledge declined significantly as did self-reports of risky behaviors.

To test the effectiveness of a program to reduce intrapersonal pressure to drink, smoke, or use drugs by developing general personal competence as well as teaching students tactics for resisting pro-use interpersonal pressure, pre- and post-test data from 1,185 randomly assigned, suburban New York, seventh grade students were analyzed (Botvin et al., 1984b). The educational program contained cognitive, decision-making, anxiety-coping, social skills, and self-improvement components. Some sections of the class were taught either by peer leaders (tenth or eleventh graders) or by regular teachers. The peer-led sections exhibited significantly greater drinking knowledge and antidrinking attitudes than did either the teacher-led or the control sections. The peer-led groups similarly consumed significantly less than did those in teacher-led or control groups. Thus, the program was only effective when taught by peer leaders.

Beam (1981) investigated possible changes in alcohol related knowledge, attitudes, and behaviors of the 27 students enrolled in a university alcohol education program. Analysis of pre- and post-test results revealed a significant increase in knowledge, but not in attitudes or behaviors.

Goodstadt and colleagues (1982) evaluated two series of ten self-contained alcohol education lessons. One series was for seventh and eighth graders; the other was for ninth and tenth graders. Eight elementary and eight secondary schools from one of the largest Canadian urban public school systems participated in the assessment. Schools had either experimental or control classes. Over 1,600 students received pre- and post-tests, which were matched by means of unique code numbers and removable name labels. In the elementary school study, experimental students were found to increase in alcohol knowledge significantly more than control students. There were no significant differences in attitudes and virtually no differences in behaviors. In the secondary school study, experimental students also exhibited significantly greater gains in knowledge. However, male drinkers exposed to the program became significantly more pro alcohol than those in the control group. Abstainers—those who reported that they usually did not drink—exposed to the program decreased their level of consumption. Summarizing multivariate analyses, the investigators (Goodstadt et al., 1982, pp. 365–366) asserted that:

These results, although complicated, present a consistent pattern: (1) Recipients of the experimental program improved their knowledge about alcohol. (2) Changes in drinking status were positive (i.e., from use to nonuse) among drinkers and were greater than among abstainers. (Abstainers, of course, could change their status only by shifting form nonuse to use, which occurred less frequently.) (3) Abstainers in the experimental group were more likely than their controls to report not drinking after the program. (4) Drinkers in the experimental group, more than their controls, tended to report drinking in the week following the program.

A peer intervention program was developed (McPherson et al., 1983) to motivate and provide skills for high school age youth to intervene in the drinking and driving behavior of their peers. McKnight and McPherson (1986, p. 340) explained that:

During the program, students participate in role-playing activities designed to show them that it is possible to intervene and to feel comfortable doing so. Students first act out prepared scenarios and roles. Later they devise their own scenarios for role playing. Student discussion is used throughout, to help clarify information and to reinforce important ideas. The program required nine hours: one hour of the information presentation and eight hours of role playing.

An evaluation of the program's effectiveness involved 667 students in five Rhode Island high schools, some received the peer intervention program and the others received the regular safety school program. Pre-tests, post-tests, and follow-up tests included measures of knowledge, attitude, and behavior (i.e., self-reported intervention). Both the peer intervention program and the conventional alcohol safety program led to significant increases in knowledge, but neither led to significant changes in attitudes. The peer intervention program was associated with significant increases in self-reported intervention.

Over 700 students participated in a study of alcohol education at five Pennsylvania community colleges (Meacci, 1990). Experimental students were enrolled in alcohol awareness courses while controls were enrolled in other courses. Data were collected through a pre-test, post-test and follow-up test. They revealed that the courses were associated with significantly increased alcohol knowledge between pre- and post-testing, but not with changes in attitude during that period. Importantly, the experimental groups scored significantly higher on negative consequences on the three month follow-up test. Thus, it was counterproductive.

DeJong (1987) conducted an evaluation of DARE's effectiveness on alcohol knowledge, attitudes, and behaviors of seventh graders. Two hundred eighty-eight students from four Los Angeles junior high schools who reported having completed a full semester of DARE were compared to 310 students who reported not having had the course. Pre-tests were not administered. Data from the post-test indicated no difference in drug knowledge or attitudes between DARE and non DARE exposed students. However, those who completed the course reported significantly lower consumption of alcohol.

The effectiveness of three educational approaches for the prevention of adolescent alcohol use was investigated by Schlegel and colleagues (1984), who compared (1) a factual approach, (2) a facts plus values clarification, and (3) a facts plus values clarification plus guided decision-making approach. (See Schlegel et al., 1984, pp. 412–419 for a detailed description). Three hundred twelve students, who served as either experimental or control subjects, completed a pre-test, a post-test and a six month follow-up test to identify changes in knowledge, attitudes, and behavior. Following exposure to the educational programs, the factual group exhibited significantly greater increases than the control group. There were no significant differences in attitudes between any groups. However, the factual group tended to drink less frequently and in reduced quantity compared to the other educational groups and the control group. In no instances did the values clarification or decision-making groups differ significantly from the control group.

The effectiveness of an alcohol education program based on social learning theory and taught to eighth grade students was examined by Theurer (1987). One hundred male and female eighth graders from three northeastern suburban Catholic schools participated in the study. The alcohol education program was taught in one classroom in each of two schools but not taught in a third school. Information on alcohol knowledge, attitudes, and behaviors was collected by means of a pre-test, post-test, and six month follow-up test. Significant results included an increase in knowledge in the treatment groups compared to the control group, although this increase was not maintained at the six month follow-up. Attitudes toward alcohol remained unchanged in the treatment group, whereas the control group's attitudes became significantly less anti-alcohol. There was no significant change in drinking behavior.

Carl (1983) assessed the effects of the Moving Through Adolescence with Confidence Curriculum on substance knowledge, attitudes, and behaviors. The curriculum is an affective, psychosocial approach that attempts to enhance self-esteem, improve decision making skills, encourage goal setting, teach stress reduction techniques, and improve communication skills. Seventy-eight students at a small, northeastern Indiana high school were assigned, although not randomly, to two experimental and one control group. Analysis of pre- and post-test results revealed virtually no program impact. However, alcohol use was lower in one of the experimental groups after the program.

A course for junior high school students emphasizing decision making was assessed for effectiveness by Schaps and his colleagues (1982). "Although factual information was provided in the course, most of the class time was spent: (a) teaching Lasswell's framework for understanding motives and needs (Lasswell and Rubenstein, 1966), (b) teaching a systematic decision-making process, (c) examining the personal and social consequences of drug use decisions, and (d) identifying alternatives to drug use in various choice situations" (Moskowitz et al., 1984a, p. 45). In the study conducted at a suburban school in northern California, 18 social studies classes were paired on the basis of grade level (seventh or eighth grade), ability level (low or heterogeneous), and student pre-test data on current use of alcohol, tobacco, and marijuana. One class in each pair was assigned to the experimental condition while the other served as a control. A total of 500 students were enrolled in the experimental (N=244) and control classes (N=256). Results revealed that very few significant differences occurred among the numerous knowledge, attitude and behavioral variables. Compared to the controls, the seventh grade experimental girls had greater drug knowledge and were less involved in the use of alcohol.

One year later, the investigators (Moskowitz et al., 1984a) conducted a follow-up study by readministering the post-test. Fewer significant differences occurred at follow-up than expected by chance. Thus, the few immediate effects did not endure over time. A third follow-up revealed similarly disappointing results (Moskowitz et al., 1984b).

Because of these negative findings, the course was modified and lengthened. All seventh grade students at one school received the revised drug education program, many of the teachers received in-service training to increase their sensitivity to both the cognitive and affective needs of students, and the next year about one-third of the students participated in "alternatives" activities providing services to others (tutoring or operating a school store). Students at another school served as a comparison group. It was found that the two year program increased drug knowledge among students in the treatment school relative to those in the control school, presumably due to the drug education. However, there was no impact of teacher training on student attitudes nor of student participation in alternative activities on alcohol attitudes or behaviors. The investigators concluded that the teacher training and alternative activity strategy were ineffective (Moskowitz et al., 1983, p. 401). A second study of the impact on attitudes and behaviors of the same alternative activities among eighth and ninth graders similarly found the strategy to be ineffective (Malvin et al., 1985).

The impact of an educational program on fraternity members was examined by comparing results of pre- and post-tests (Conyne, 1984). Comparison of mean scores and percentages between the experimental and control groups indicated that "the alcohol education treatment produced either no differences or quite subtle ones, with the exception of an obvious increase in factual information about alcohol." The investigators continued that "In the latter instance, members of the alcohol education treatment group improved their correct responses to alcohol information questions from 58 percent to 96 percent (pre- to post-tests), though control group members' responses remained unchanged at 65 percent to 64 percent (pre- to post-tests). That knowledge increases lead to attitudinal or behavioral changes, however seems unlikely" (Conyne, 1984, p. 527).

The Alcohol Misuse Prevention Study (AMPS) is based on a social skills approach; its focus is on teaching the acquisition of behavioral skills to resist pressures to misuse alcohol (Dielman et al., 1987). To test its effectiveness, 5,680 fifth and sixth grade students from 213 Michigan classrooms were randomly assigned by school building to one of three experimental conditions: treatment, treatment plus booster, and control. In addition to pre-testing, there was also post-testing at the end of the first school year in which AMPS was presented, as well as follow-up testing at the end of the two following school years. Exposure to the AMPS program was associated with a significant increase in knowledge about alcohol at post-test (two months after the course) and the first follow-up (14 months after the course). Those who received booster sessions exhibited significantly greater knowledge than either those who received only the course or no instruction. The program demonstrated no effect on either alcohol use or misuse (Dielman et al., 1987; Campanelli et al., 1989). Subsequent analyses indicated that the program was effective in reducing the rate of increase of alcohol use and misuse among sixth grade students who entered the study with prior supervised (as well as unsupervised) alcohol use, but for no other category of student (Dielman et al., 1989; Dielman et al., 1992).

Simpson (1979) compared the effectiveness of a cognitive and a cognitive/affective approach to alcohol education on the knowledge, attitudes and behavior of college students. One experimental group received the cognitive approach, while the other received the cognitive/affective approach. These two groups, as well as a control group, were administered a pre-test and a post-test. When compared to the control group, both experimental groups demonstrated significant increases in knowledge and attitudes; there were no differences between the experimental groups. There were also no significant differences in behavior between the control and the experimental group or between the two experimental groups.

A ten week program of alcohol education was evaluated among fourth and fifth grade students in the United Kingdom (Heaney, 1984). The participants were pupils at seven different secondary schools; four schools were assigned to the experimental group and four to the control group. All received a pre-test, a post-test and a three month follow-up test to assess alcohol knowledge, attitudes, and behaviors. The experimental group exhibited a significant increase in knowledge and a significant change in attitude toward alcohol, neither of which persisted for as long as three months. The only other significant change was a decrease in frequency in drinking in the *control* group, which did not persist for three months.

Not easily categorized elsewhere is Fischer's (1990) study of the effectiveness of three instructional approaches (traditional, values clarification, and disease concept) among college students in which the post-test responses of 267 students were analyzed. The subjects had completed courses using the various approaches at three colleges on the Pacific coast. There was no control group. Analysis of variance indicated that there was no significant difference among the three instructional approaches regarding students' knowledge about alcohol. However, the values clarification approach resulted in significantly less accepting attitudes among women about alcohol use and abuse.

Similarly the effectiveness of "an innovative, theory-based, peer-focused college drug education academic course" in modifying students' perceived level of risk associated with the use of alcohol was evaluated by administering pre- and post-tests to 110 students enrolled in the course and to 95 students in two control classes (Gonzalez, 1989; 1990, p. 446). Code numbers known only to the investigator made it possible to match pre- and post-tests; 96 matched questionnaires were obtained from the experimental group and 80 from the control group. The drug education course did not produce an increase in perceived risk from using alcohol.

RESPONSIBLE-USE PROGRAMS

Responsible-use programs are demonstrably more effective than no-use programs. Being discouraged by federal policy, there are relatively few responsible-use programs and few studies of those programs. Only one study has examined the impact of such a program on knowledge only; it found a significant increase in alcohol knowledge. No study has examined solely attitudes. Of the three studies of behavior, two (67%) found a significant positive change while one found mixed results.

Twelve studies have examined the impact of responsible use programs on the three variables of knowledge, attitudes, and behaviors. Four (33%) of these report significant positive impact on all three variables, two report no impact, while six (50%) report mixed findings. Eleven investigations examine the impact of such programs on two variables (knowledge and attitude, knowledge and behavior, or attitude and behavior). Three of the eleven (27%) report significant positive impact on both variables examined while eight report mixed (although generally favorable) findings.

Knowledge Increased by Responsible-Use Programs

One study assessed the effects of alcohol education on knowledge only. Three hundred thirty-four students in 13 elementary schools in South Carolina received instruction in the "Here's Looking at You, Two" program while students in two other schools constituted the control group (Mahaffey, 1988). All students were pre- and post-tested. The resulting data indicated a significant increase in knowledge by the experimental group and by one of the two control groups. The second control group exhibited an increase in knowledge that was not significant. However, the experimental group's increase was significantly greater than the combined control group's increase.

Behavior Improved in Two of Three Studies

Three studies have examined the impact of alcohol education on behavior only, with generally positive results. A responsible-use health development program in Australia was designed, among other things, "to educate for use rather than abuse" (Homel et al., 1981, p. 269). Its effectiveness was studied among 1,850 experimental students from kindergarten through twelfth grade compared to 1,350 control students in kindergarten through twelfth grade. Measures of health behaviors were developed for students in fifth grade, sixth grade, junior high (grades 7–10), and senior high (11 and 12 grades). Each questionnaire covered basically the same content, the major differences being the level of difficulty and detail of the questions. However, only secondary students answered questions regarding alcohol consumption. Students completed the instrument before the curriculum was introduced to the experimental group and again two years later. The results demonstrated that:

there has been a large and highly significant change in the patterns of heavy ("daily") drinking amongst the boys in each school ($X^2 = 31.246$, p<.001), such that the control school has shown a significant increase and the experimental school has shown a significant drop. This change is also reflected in a significant decrease in the number of boys drinking at all in the experimental school and an increase in the control school ($X^2 = 8.003$, p<.005). The changes in the daily drinking rates of the girls are also significant, if not as large as the boys. There has been a drop in the number of heavy ("daily") drinkers in the experimental school and an increase at the control school ($X^2 = 4.389$, p<.05). (Homel et al., 1981, p. 268)

The authors stressed that "These highly significant drops in alcohol consumption do in fact contradict the general regional trend for increasing consumption rates amongst these age groups. This result becomes even more important when it is realized that alcohol abuse was a perceived local health problem which was specifically addressed within the context of the health/personal development programme" (Homel et al, 1981, p. 269).

Wragg (1986) assessed an educational program based on the philosophy that "The goal of developing responsible drug use may be preferable to promoting abstinence" (p. 285). An experimental group of 31 students and a control group of

33 students aged ten to twelve completed a pre-test and then a post-test three and one-half years later. The researcher found that:

Subjects from the experimental group used [alcohol and] drugs less frequently and to a lesser degree. The preference towards more responsible use on the part of the experimental group is also supported by the self-report measures regarding the after-effects of drinking alcohol. It may well be that drug education programmes cannot prevent drug use per se but they may well have a valuable contribution to make in the development of attitudes and behavior consistent with responsible and moderate drug use. From the evidence presented in this study it would appear that drug education programmes that choose abstinence as their major goal are likely to regard drug education as completely wasted; it would be more realistic to focus on the development of responsible drug use as the preferred goal of drug education. (Wragg, 1986, p. 292)

An evaluation of a responsible use program involved comparing pre- and post-test scores at two schools in Pennsylvania; one used the curriculum for eighth grade students and one did not. While frequency of drinking did not decrease among experimental students, drinking to become drunk and quantity consumed per occasion did.

Knowledge, Attitudes, and Behaviors Changed by Responsible-Use Programs

Campus Alcohol Policies and Education (CAPE) is a program for college freshmen that uses two approaches—education and policy—to reduce the excessive and/or inappropriate use of alcohol:

The education component involves the transmission of information about appropriate and inappropriate uses of alcohol for university students, all focusing on the four potential problems: when drinking becomes drunkenness; drinking and health; drinking and driving; drinking and academics. The information is disseminated through booklets mailed to each first year student, posters, print media advertisements, and residence presentations. The policy component focuses on the implementation of specific strategies, by tavern managers and administration, to make it more difficult for students to drink excessively or to suffer the negative consequences of such drinking. (Gliksman et al., 1987, p. iv)

The major goals of the program are:

1. To increase students' knowledge about low-risk drinking behavior;
2. to change attitudes favorable to selecting and maintaining low-risk drinking practices; and
3. to promote the adoption of low-risk drinking practices. (Gliksman et al., 1987, p. 2)

More specifically, the personal moderation message was designed to persuade students to avoid four risky drinking behaviors:

1. High average levels of consumption;
2. drinking and driving;
3. drinking to drunkenness; and
4. drinking before undertaking academic activities. (Gliksman et al., 1987, p. 2)

For those students who chose to drink (the program emphasized that the decision to abstain is also a responsible and desirable one), the following prescriptions were stressed:

1. Drink no more than one drink per hour and no more than four drinks per occasion;
2. consume seven drinks or fewer per week;
3. don't drink if driving; and
4. don't drink when studying. (Gliksman et al., 1987, p. 4)

To assess the impact of the program on student attitudes and behaviors, pre- and post-test scores were analyzed. The findings are arranged in terms of knowledge, attitudes, and behaviors.

Knowledge. Although both experimental and control groups increased in alcohol knowledge, experimental students demonstrated a significantly greater increase.

Attitude. Numerous scales measured a diversity of attitudes. Experimental students decreased in their intended drinking frequency whereas control students increased in theirs. Both experimental and control students became less censorious toward drunkenness, but control students did so to a greater degree. Experimental students increased their feelings that drinking and driving for themselves was bad, while control students decreased their feelings in this regard. Experimental students developed more negative attitudes toward drinking and driving by anyone, whereas control students exhibited no change over time. Experimental students increased in negative attitude toward alcohol use and studying or attending class (i.e., an attitude against combining alcohol with academics) whereas control students' attitude became more accepting of combining them. Experimental students dramatically increased in positive, accepting attitudes toward abstinence whereas control students became more rejecting of abstinence. Experimental students did not express an increased intention to get drunk in the coming school year whereas control students did. Experimental students showed a significant decrease in intention to use alcohol with academic activities (i.e., prior to studying, while studying, or prior to an exam) whereas control students showed a slight increase in those intentions. Experimental students increased in intention to use less alcohol in the future whereas control students decreased in that intention.

Behavior. Frequency of alcohol use remained stable among experimental students whereas it increased significantly among the controls. Increased frequency is the typical pattern among college students; it appears that the educational program was successful in maintaining it at pre-college levels. The experimental students decreased in weekly alcohol consumption whereas control students demonstrated a significant increase. Experimentals demonstrated a dramatic increase in responsible behavior toward alcohol use while the controls revealed no change. Experimental students did not demonstrate as great an increase in drinking problems as the control group. Thus, it appears that CAPE had a moderating effect. In short, CAPE was successful in increasing alcohol knowledge, changing attitudes, and—most importantly—positively influencing actual drinking behavior.

A study of the effects of a controlled usage alcohol education program on college students involved four sections of exercise and health at a midwestern university (Portnoy, 1980). Two sections of the course constituted the experimental groups while two other sections constituted the control groups. The alcohol education program consisted of two 50 minute lectures on alcohol use. The Responsible Alcohol Use Inventory was administered during the second week (pre-test), fourth week (post-test), and ninth week (second or follow-up post-test). The inventory attempts to assess how responsible an individual's drinking practices are through seven Likert-type items such as "Whenever I drink alcoholic beverages I sip rather than gulp my drink" and "Whenever I drink alcoholic beverages, I also eat food or snack foods such as pretzels, potato chips, etc." (Portnoy, 1980, p. 188). The researcher suggested the desirability of using the educational program with students exhibiting non-responsible drinking patterns. "In the meantime, the program is effective for populations with current responsible drinking patterns in that it increased alcohol knowledge levels, reinforced desirable attitudes and beliefs, and positively affected [i.e., lowered] beer consumption patterns" (Portnoy, 1980, p. 193).

The purpose of Claydon's (1982) study was to assess the effects of participation in alcohol education designed to increase responsible decision making and reduce irresponsible behaviors and negative consequences associated with college students' use of alcohol. Fraternities and sororities at a California state university campus were randomly assigned to treatment and control group conditions. A three month alcohol education program to increase responsible use of alcohol was developed by student representatives from the experimental chapters with assistance from the campus Alcohol Awareness Program. The alcohol education program included drinking and driving demonstrations, facts and issues flyers, films and discussions on alcohol, a nonalcohol sporting and social event, and informal workshops on alcohol topics. The control chapters received the flyers and were eligible to attend program activities. An anonymous self-report survey consisting of demographic items and 129 items of knowledge, attitudes, and behaviors concerning alcohol was randomly administered as a pre-test to half the fraternity and sorority subjects. After the program, it was administered to all the fraternity and sorority subjects. No significant differences were found between experimental and control groups at pre-test. However, post-tested subjects in the treatment condition reported significantly higher levels of knowledge, responsible attitudes, and responsible behaviors than did control group subjects.

The Campus Alcohol Information Center at the University of Florida conducted research to determine if "knowledge about alcohol and responsible attitudes toward alcohol can be affected so as to increase the likelihood of specific alcohol related behavior which would be conducive to a reduction of alcohol related problems among a specific population" (Gonzalez, 1982, pp. 3–4). The center examined alcohol knowledge, attitudes, and behavior among 499 college student drinkers enrolled at six different universities in the southeast and found a significant inverse relationship between responsible attitudes toward alcohol and the incidence of drinking problems. Given the relationship found between responsible attitudes and behavior, Gonzalez (1980) sought to increase responsible attitudes among college students. Sixty-three students were randomly assigned to the experimental group; the same number were assigned to the control group. The experimental group was given a four hour alcohol education module designed to promote responsible alcohol attitudes. It made use of peer leaders, audiovisual materials, value clarification exercises, and small group techniques. Students were pre-tested with all three of the above measures, then post-tested immediately after the educational workshops for knowledge and responsible attitudes. Finally, three months later they were given a follow-up post-test with all three measures. The program significantly increased the degree of responsibility in attitudes and the level of alcohol knowledge, and these changes persisted for at least three months. However, there was no difference between experimental and control groups in drinking problems.

These findings led to a follow-up study by Rozelle (1980), in which he examined the relative effectiveness of an experiential and a cognitive approach in teaching knowledge and responsible attitudes regarding alcohol and in reducing drinking problems. These variables were assessed with a pre-test, post-test, and three month follow-up post-test. Students were randomly assigned to ten small group discussion sections; five used a cognitive curriculum and five used an experiential approach. A control group consisted of students randomly selected from two elective courses. In the experiential course, students participated in a responsible cocktail party and visited drinking establishments and alcohol treatment centers. The experiential and cognitive approaches both produced significantly higher levels of responsible attitudes than the control group, which persisted for at least three months. The two approaches were also equally effective in producing significant increases in knowledge, which also persisted for at least three months. While there were no immediately significant differences in negative consequences from drinking, three months later both the experiential and cognitive groups experienced significantly fewer drinking problems than did the control group.

Several studies have obtained mixed results regarding alcohol knowledge, attitudes, and behavior. For example, Miller (1982) compared the effectiveness of the traditional and the responsible-use approaches to alcohol education for college students. The 254 students who participated in the study were enrolled in six one-credit health education courses at a large Pennsylvania university. Two of the sections were on human sexuality and served as the control group. Two of the remaining sections received the traditional approach and two received the responsible-use approach to alcohol education. All students were pre- and post-tested for alcohol knowledge, attitudes, and behaviors. Significant pre-course to post-course differences in knowledge were found between the responsible-use, traditional, and control groups. Students in the responsible-use groups gained in knowledge more than did those in the traditional or control group and students in the traditional groups increased more than did students in the control group. There were no significant changes in alcohol attitudes. Both experimental groups experienced greater changes in drinking patterns than did the control group. "The responsible-use group experienced a decrease in consequences resulting from the use of beverage alcohol, while the traditional and control groups experienced an increase in consequences resulting from the use of beverage alcohol, a difference significant at the .001 level. When the responsible-use group and the traditional group were compared, a significant (.001) difference was obtained" (Miller, 1982, p. 85).

The effects of three educational methodologies (implicit instruction, explicit instruction, and values clarification) were investigated by Robinson, 1980, 1981). Implicit instruction consisted of class lectures that provided factual information only. No conclusions were drawn for the students and no recommendations were made. Explicit instruction consisted of lectures providing factual information, followed by stated conclusions and specific recommendations. Values clarification instruction consisted of class lectures similar to the content of the above treatments. However, neither conclusions nor recommendations were made. Instead, values clarification strategies were presented. Each teaching methodology was presented for four 50 minute class sessions to students attending college level general health classes. Pre-tests were administered during the class period before the educational methodologies were begun in the randomly assigned treatment sections and in a control class. A second control group was used to identify any reactive effects from testing. One week after the last treatment session, the post-test was administered. Follow-up data were collected three weeks after the post-test data were collected. The questionnaire assessed alcohol knowledge, attitudes, and behaviors. The investigator found that all treatment groups exhibited significantly greater increases in knowledge than did the control group, and the explicit instruction approach produced changes in attitudes or behavior.

The CASPAR (Cambridge and Somerville Program for Alcohol Rehabilitation) education prevention program for third grade through twelfth grade, "Decisions about Drinking," was assessed among several schools in Georgia (DiCicco et al., 1984). The results of testing over time suggest significant increases in knowledge but less consistent changes in attitudes. The investigators observed that the results suggested that there may be a behavioral impact of instruction in the form of reduced alcohol misuse among teenagers, although if there is, it requires intensive and repeated exposure and can be demonstrated in these data only among younger students while they remain in junior high school. While such results may be viewed as less supportive than the original experiment, they do suggest that alcohol education remains an effective prevention strategy (DiCicco et al., 1984, p. 160).

A sample of 214 students at a technical college in Australia participated in a study of alcohol knowledge, attitudes, and behaviors (Manley Drug Education and Counselling Centre, 1987). Classes were randomly assigned to treatment and non treatment conditions. In addition to pre- and post-testing, follow-up testing occurred one month after the post-test. Positive changes were found in knowledge but not in attitudes or behavior.

The "Here's Looking at You" alcohol education program was also evaluated in a large North Carolina school system for its effectiveness in increasing alcohol knowledge, changing attitudes (undifferentiated-premature attitudes, reward-associated attitudes, and health-related attitudes), and changing actual drinking behavior (Kim, 1988). About 900 students in fourth grade through sixth grade participated in the HLAY program while about 135 in the same grade levels were in the control group. Students in both the experimental and control groups were matched for the pre- and post-tests using a special identification code uniquely assigned to each student. Results indicated that the experimental group increased in knowledge, but its gain was less than that exhibited by the control group. There were few attitudinal improvements among the HYAY group and none in actual drinking behavior.

For his doctoral research, Eakin (1984) evaluated the peer education component of the Total Awareness Program developed at Pennsylvania State University. Pre- and post- tests assessed alcohol knowledge, attitudes, and behaviors. There was no program impact on alcohol knowledge or drinking patterns. While responsible drinking attitudes improved for women, they declined among men.

Observing virtually no impact on knowledge, attitudes, or behavior was a longitudinal assessment of the "Here's Looking at You" curriculum (Hopkins et al., 1988) with 6,808 students in fourth grades through twelve in five Pacific Northwest school districts (Hopkins et al., 1988). Pre-tests, post-tests and follow-up tests were linked by means of a student specific unique nonsensitive identification code. The investigators concluded that the curriculum had little impact on students.

Eighty-four nonalcohol dependent college students at a large state university volunteered for a study to determine the effects of a five hour moderate drinking skill training course (Kennedy, 1989). The behavioral self-management program involved meeting one hour per week in small groups for five weeks and provided a combination of alcohol information and self-control skill training. Control group members received no training and both groups completed the same outcome instruments at immediate and long term follow-up. Subjects were assessed on alcohol knowledge, alcohol attitudes and three measures of drinking behavior (total number of drinks, average blood alcohol, and peak blood alcohol) derived from self-report retrospective drinking diaries completed both at immediate and long-term follow-up. At the end of the training sessions, there were significant differences between the experimental and control groups on knowledge, average blood alcohol content (BAC), and peak BAC. Five months later, the average BAC and peak BAC were no longer significantly different from the control group. Both the treatment and control groups showed a reduction in the total number of drinks consumed. This reduction in drinking was also reflected in reduced average BAC and peak BAC for both groups. As the study's author correctly notes:

The fact that both the treatment and control groups showed a similar reduction in drinking behavior implicates non-treatment factors as agents in this reduction. It also underlines the importance of using a control group in outcome studies since a contrast with baseline data alone may have resulted in attributing this effect to treatment. (Kennedy, 1989, p. 144)

Knowledge and Attitudes Usually Changed by Responsible-Use Programs

Four studies have investigated the impact of alcohol education of knowledge and attitude, but not on behavior. Reporting a positive impact on knowledge and attitude was a study of a CASPAR alcohol prevention curriculum (Stover, 1984). One hundred and sixty-eight ninth through twelfth graders in a small town Wisconsin high school completed pre- and post-tests. There was no control group in this investigation, which found a significant positive change in alcohol knowledge and attitudes between pre- and post-testing.

A basic objective of the Stanford D-E-C-I-D-E drug education curriculum is to encourage responsible use of alcohol for those who choose to drink. D-E-C-I-D-E is an acronym for *define* the problem, *explore* the alternatives, *consider* the influence of others and the consequences of a decision, *invite* outside opinion, *determine* a course of action, and *evaluate* the outcome of the decision. This decision-making curriculum emphasizes group interaction and addresses such topics as peer pressure, value development, problem-solving, self-image, and attitudes toward authority. An analysis of the curriculum's impact on the alcohol knowledge and attitudes of junior high school students was conducted with 27 eighth grade students in a classroom randomly selected from a public school in southern Illinois (Gray, 1984). Responses of the pre- and post-test indicated a significant increase in knowledge as well as a significant change in attitudes in the desired (i.e., responsible) direction.

The Alaska Council on Prevention of Alcohol and Drug Abuse, Inc. (1982) conducted a study of "Here's Looking at You, Two" with 1,594 students in 30 schools throughout the state. Students were categorized by educational level (fourth grade, fifth grade, sixth grade, and junior high) and by community category (urban, hub city, and village). All were given pre- and post-tests to measure alcohol and drug knowledge and attitudes. Students demonstrated significant increases in knowledge except for those who attended junior high schools located in villages. However, the data regarding attitudes were inconsistent; both significant increases and decreases were found.

Green and Kelley (1989) evaluated the effectiveness of "Here's Looking at You, Two" in a Pennsylvania demonstration project. One thousand six hundred ninety-eight treatment students and 1,005 control students at elementary and middle schools in five Indiana school districts participated in a study of the program's effectiveness in increasing knowledge and changing attitudes regarding alcohol. All data comparing experimentals and controls revealed a statistically significant increase in knowledge about drugs and alcohol attributable to the effects of the educational program. However, it had little impact on alcohol attitudes.

Knowledge and Behaviors More Effectively Impacted by Responsible-Use Approach

Several studies have examined the impact of alcohol education on knowledge and behavior, but not on attitudes. For example, an alcohol education program designed to reduce the use and abuse of alcohol among elementary school pupils was evaluated in 213 fifth and sixth grade classrooms in six Michigan school districts (Dielman et al., 1986). A total of 5,635 students were randomly assigned by school building to one of three conditions: treatment, treatment plus booster, and control. Students were post-tested at the end of the school year in which the prevention program was presented. Comparison of pre- and post-test results revealed that experimental students significantly increased in alcohol "knowledge" (for example, that "alcohol commercials brainwash people to want to be like the people in the ads"). In spite of such content, the program is described by the researchers as responsible use in nature. There were no differences between experimental and control students in the use of alcohol or in problems resulting from drinking alcohol.

Exposure to the program was associated with a significant increase in knowledge at the first follow-up testing 14 months after the course. Those who received booster sessions exhibited significantly greater knowledge than those who received only the course or no instruction. The program did not demonstrate an effect on alcohol use or misuse (Dielman et al., 1987). However, subsequent analyses of data collected 26 months after the program revealed that it was effective in reducing alcohol use among sixth grade students who entered the study with prior unsupervised use of alcohol (Dielman et al., 1989; Shope et al., 1992).

Another study was conducted targeting sixth grade students, because a group of pupils at that level had shown both cognitive and behavioral benefits from the program. For this study:

the curriculum was expanded and enhanced by adding more sessions, role playing, refutation of common expectations for alcohol use, norm-setting, and by having students use their knowledge and experience to guide problem-solving and decision-making about alcohol use. Follow-up seventh and eighth grade sessions were developed, providing students with opportunities to practice resistance strategies as they experienced increasing social pressure to use alcohol. This expanded curriculum provided students with enhanced rationale and positive peer support for resisting pressure to use and misuse alcohol. (Shope et al., 1994, p. 160)

Thirty-five elementary and middle school buildings were matched (by achievement test scores, proportion receiving free and reduced lunches, and ethnicity of sixth grade students) within districts, then assigned randomly to experimental or control conditions. All sixth graders were pre-tested at the beginning of the school year and then post-tested in the spring of their sixth, seventh, and eighth grades. The curriculum was implemented in the treatment schools in the winter of the students' sixth, seventh, and eighth grades. Results indicated that treatment group students achieved significantly higher knowledge scores than did control students. The curriculum also led to a significantly lower rate of increase in alcohol misuse among those who had used alcohol unsupervised by adults (Shope et al., 1994).

The effectiveness of a peer-led versus a staff-led college alcohol education program was assessed among 37 students who were randomly assigned to a peer-led or staff-led treatment; there was no control group (Kuehn, 1991). Students were given a pre-test, a post-test and a follow-up test fifteen days after completing the program. The results indicated that those in the staff-led group scored significantly higher on knowledge at both testings after the intervention. However, there was no impact of either approach on drinking behavior.

To assess the effects of teaching specific guidelines for alcohol consumption on knowledge and behavioral intent, a convenience sample of 87 volunteer subjects was selected from three classes at a southeastern university (Jackson et al., 1989). One class received the standard alcohol education curriculum, another received that curriculum plus consumption guidelines, while a third received no alcohol education. Pre- and post-test data revealed that the experimental classes experienced significantly greater increases in knowledge compared to the control group but not from each other.

Attitudes and Behaviors Improved by Responsible-Use Programs

Two studies analyzed the effect of alcohol education on attitude and behavior, but not on knowledge. "Tip It Lightly, Alcohol Awareness Week" used a variety of activities at a large midwestern university. During the awareness week:

Students voluntarily attended sessions on communication, alcohol and driving, sexuality, stress management, and other topics related to alcohol issues and concerns. Pledges of responsible drinking were collected at several locations on campus. Residence halls competed for awards in the areas of non-alcoholic alternatives and number of pledges of responsible drinking. Alternatives to alcohol were emphasized during such campus activities as dances, debates, and non-alcoholic happy hours. (Chen et al., 1982, p. 126)

One thousand students were randomly selected by computer from the approximately 8,500 students enrolled at the university. Surveys were mailed to the subjects with return envelopes provided. Return rate was 55 percent for the pre-program survey and 45 percent for the post-program survey. Pre- and post-test comparisons were made for the total sample and for those who had participated in the alcohol education program. Some improvement in attitudes were found among those who participated in the program. More importantly, participants reported significant decreases in heavy drinking and episodes of intoxication per week. Both groups reported fewer hangovers and less nausea and vomiting from drinking, but only participants reported less often damaging property. The authors concluded that "for those subjects who participated in the program, there was a significant improvement in their drinking attitudes and behaviors" (Chen et al., 1982, p. 126; Chen and Bosch, 1987).

All eighth grade students in twelve diverse schools in Pennsylvania were exposed to the "Here's Looking at You Two" program. All eighth graders at two additional schools served as the control group. Pre- and post-test comparisons revealed that there was no difference between experimental and control groups in willingness to use beer and liquor (no questions were asked regarding wine). But while there was no difference between the groups in the proportions consuming these beverages, intoxication was significantly less frequent among those exposed to the program. The investigators noted that "The reductions in self-reported drunkenness suggest that the experimental group students became more moderate in their drinking patterns. This is especially important in that frequency of drinking did not decrease, but apparently amount per occasion did decrease" (Swisher et al., 1985, p. 116).

Two studies are difficult to categorize elsewhere. Allison and his colleagues (Allison et al., 1990) compared the effects of intensive staff development, in-service training, and no in-service training on fifth graders' alcohol knowledge and behavioral intentions. The data were collected as part of an evaluation of "Drug Abuse Prevention Project—an Education Resource," a joint project of an Ontario Board of Education and the Addiction Research Foundation. One experimental group consisted of 92 students in four classrooms whose teachers had received intensive staff development on the curriculum. Another consisted of 107 students in five classrooms whose teachers had received brief in-service training. A control group of 67 pupils in three classrooms had teachers who received curriculum guidelines only. A questionnaire was administered to all students at the beginning and end of the school year and revealed that differential teacher training was not associated with major differences in knowledge. The investigators (Allison et al., 1990, p. 40) reported that "The only statistically significant differences between groups were at both pre- and post-test on the proportion intending to drink alcohol, if offered. There were significant differences at post-test between those exposed to intensive staff development versus in-service training, and between those exposed to intensive staff development vs. the control group."

Traditionally, alcohol education research has focused on group outcomes data and has not examined the possibility of differential effectiveness among different categories of students. However, one study (Pipher and Rivers, 1982) examined this phenomenon among 67 junior high students who were assigned to the four health class sections employed in the study. Assignment was made by the school administration based on which section best fit their schedules. Two sections were experimental, in which a decision-making alcohol course was taught over a seven week period, while two were control section in which no alcohol education occurred. One experimental and one control section completed a 79 item research questionnaire before the experimental course began and filled out weekly drinking records each week. After completion of the alcohol course, all four sections completed the questionnaire. Two months later, all sections were administered critical items from the questionnaire as a follow-up. Analysis of difference scores between pre- and post-testing (including the two month follow-up) revealed that only some positive results endured for an additional two months (Pipher and

Rivers, 1982). However, it was discovered that the course had positive effects for some students, but negative effects for others. Students who had firsthand knowledge of the problems of alcohol abuse of a friend or relative experienced more positive effects. The course also seemed to be more effective for students whose social groups and activities involved less deviant behavior.

CONCLUSION

It is obvious that responsible-use alcohol education programs are demonstrably more successful than are no-use programs. It is important to note that, "when alcohol/drug attitudes are conveyed in the alcohol curriculum, they are usually negative abstinence ones, even with so-called responsible drinking approaches" (Blom and Snoddy, 1980, p. 259). Such curricula rarely, if ever, even mention "the potentially positive aspects of alcohol, such as the evidence for reduced risk of heart problems from moderate use (Yano et al., 1977; Hennekens et al., 1979; Kozavarevic et al., 1980), alcohol's more general positive contribution to adolescent social adjustment (Demone, 1972), or the possibility that moderate use may even be associated with *safer* driving (Cohen, 1981)" (Weisheit, 1983, p. 74, emphasis in original). And even if a curriculum has a responsible use component, those who present it tend to "narrowly define the choices for teenagers' use of alcohol as abstinence vs. uncontrolled and disruptive drinking" (DiCicco et al., 1984, pp. 161–162). For teachers who know better than this:

A central problem, as Unterberger and DiCicco (1968) point out, is that the average American drinks "wet" but thinks "dry," i.e., despite the fact that most Americans drink moderately, they express strong misgivings about drinking, are apprehensive about alcohol and fear teenage alcohol use (DiCicco and Unterberger, 1977). As a result, school personnel develop the fallacious notion that if they are to undertake alcohol education, their goal must be one of abstinence or else they will encounter serious objections from the community (Kenney, 1978; Milgram, 1976; Mullin, 1968). (DiCicco et al., 1984, p. 161)

Two alcohol educators have pointed out that:

There are many reasons for the persistence of direct or implied abstinence attitudes toward drinking in educational endeavors in a society where paradoxically a preponderant majority drink alcoholic beverages. Our society's view toward drinking and alcohol continues to be ambivalent and conflicted, and is manifested in most public education efforts and social policy decisions (Anderson, 1979; Plaut, 1967, 1972; Blane, 1978). There is also conflict between and within states, government agencies, health professionals, educators, alcohol agencies, and citizens. Furthermore, the historical origin of many public school alcohol curricula was during the era of prohibition (Chafetz, 1979; Ferrier, 1964). Even if one examines the most enlightened current textbooks and educational materials on alcohol, there is a striking absence of information and discussion about an alternative, that drinking may contribute to positive qualities of life (Chafetz, 1967, 1973; Keller, 1979). We have not taken a collective position in our society that drinking behavior involves a developmental socialization process (Blane, 1978; Wilkinson, 1970). We have also missed a central goal about alcohol education—providing the necessary conditions for individual choice in responsible drinking and nondrinking behaviors. (Keller, 1979; Jessor et al., 1970; Mullin, 1968) (Blom and Snoddy, 1980, p. 259)

While there are numerous alcohol and drug education programs in the United States,

none is more prevalent than Project DARE (Drug Abuse Resistance Education). Created in 1983 by the Los Angeles Police Department and the Los Angeles Unified School District, DARE uses specially trained law enforcement officers to teach a drug use prevention curriculum in elementary schools and, more recently, in junior and senior high schools. Since its inception, DARE has been adopted by approximately 50% of local school districts nationwide, and it continues to spread rapidly. DARE is the only drug use prevention program specifically named in the 1986 Drug-Free Schools and Communities Act. Some 10% of the Drug-Free Schools and Communities Act governor's funds, which are 30% of the funds available each fiscal year for state and local programs, are set aside for programs "such as Project Drug Abuse Resistance Education," amounting to much of the program's public funding. (Ennett et al., 1994, p. 1394)

In spite of its widespread use, and the extensive time, money, and effort devoted to its success, it has not been widely evaluated. However, an analysis of DARE outcome evaluations focusing on short-term effectiveness led to the conclusion that its "effectiveness for reducing or preventing drug use behavior is small and is less than for interactive prevention programs"; its impact is "slight" and not statistically significant (Ennett et al., 1994, pp. 1394 and 1398). Very importantly, the investigators observed that "DARE's limited influence on adolescent drug use behavior contrasts with the program's popularity and prevalence. An important implication is that DARE could be taking the place of other, more beneficial drug use curricula that adolescents could be receiving" (Ennett et al., 1994, p. 1399).

Vast resources of money, personnel, time, and effort are being expended on DARE and other ineffective no-use programs because we are prisoners of political ideology. The next chapter addresses this serious problem.

4

Conclusion
and
Recommendations

The development of alcohol education programs should be based on the best scientific evidence available rather than on political ideology. Clearly, that is not current practice. The empirical evidence suggests that a socioculturally based responsible use approach would be more effective than the strict no-use approach promoted by the federal government. Unfortunately, the responsible use approach is typically misunderstood, mischaracterized and maligned. Making matters worse is the fact that inflated and otherwise deceptive statistics tend to pollute public "knowledge" and discussion about alcohol. This unfortunate situation leads to several recommendations.

POLICY SHOULD BE BASED ON SCIENCE, NOT IDEOLOGY

The important task of identifying alcohol education programs and techniques that effectively reduce the extent of alcohol abuse should be based on science and objective evidence rather than on political ideology. Any other approach to the task is totally indefensible and morally corrupt (Ross, 1987, p. 173; Heath, 1988a, 1988b; Room, 1988). After reviewing the effectiveness of alcohol education, one observer stressed that:

It would seem, therefore, that a great deal of effort (not to say time and money) has been expended in order to achieve comparatively little. If this situation is to be improved, then it is important to try to understand why it is that people have, for twenty years, continued to do something which has been repeatedly shown to have virtually no positive impact. Unterberger and DiCicco contend that sharp emotional disagreements concerning overall goals and plans of action have resulted in a neglect of promising instructional programmes. (Grant, 1982, p. 203)

Unfortunately, the problem is much more serious than mere neglect: it is the federally promoted effort to discourage the use of any and all programs other than those based on a strict abstinence ideology.

FEDERAL POLICY IS IDEOLOGICAL AND BIASED

While the Drug Free Schools and Communities Act does not mandate a no-use or even a reduction-of-consumption approach to alcohol education, the position of the Department of Education on this matter is clear—"Among the themes that should be present at *all* levels are the following: A clear and consistent message that the use of alcohol, tobacco, and other illicit drugs is unhealthy [i.e., unhealthful] and harmful" and "Curricula which advocate *responsible use* of drugs [which is explicitly described as including alcohol] should be rejected" (U.S. Department of Education, 1988, p. 10, emphases in original).

In its recommendations for selecting alcohol and drug curricula, the Department of Education urges educators to:

Look for "warning flag" phrases and concepts.

The following expressions, many of which appear frequently in pro-drug material, falsely imply that there is a safe use of mind-altering drugs: *experimental use, recreational use, social use, controlled use, responsible use, use/abuse.*

Mood-altering is a deceptive euphemism for mind-altering.

The implication of the phrase mood-altering is that only temporary feelings are involved. The fact is that mood changes are biological changes in the brain.

"There are no good or bad drugs, just improper use."

This is a popular semantic camouflage in pro-drug literature. It confuses young people and minimizes the distinct chemical differences among substances.

"The child's own decision."

Parents cannot afford to leave such hazardous choices to their children. It is the parents' responsibility to do all in their power to provide the information and the protection to assure their children a drug-free childhood and adolescence.

Be alert for contradictory messages.

Many authors give a pro-drug message then cover their tracks by including *cautions* about how to use drugs. (U.S. Department of Education, 1992, p. 28, emphases in original)

Health educators who attended the first National Conference on Drug and Alcohol Abuse Prevention sponsored by the National Institute on Alcohol Abuse and Alcoholism and the National Institute on Drug Abuse reported that they "were told to 'purge' responsible alcohol use from our minds when thinking of alcohol education curricula and content for young people, and even for adults. The philosophy behind this thinking suggests that we should not consider responsible use if, 1) our goal is drug-free youth, and 2) the drinking age is above the age of our target group; we should not provide information about responsible choices concerning alcohol or responsible drinking for those who might choose to drink when they are of legal age as this might be encouraging young people to [drink]" (Engs and Fors, 1988, p. 26).

A reduction-of-consumption writer (Horton, 1988, pp. 5–6) asserts that "We must reject the idea of teaching responsible use of alcohol; to do so is self-defeating and dangerous. Alcohol is illegal for underage people and there can be no responsible use of an illegal substance." He contends that "We must send an unambiguous message that no use of alcohol or other drugs is expected or acceptable, in any amount at any time, under any condition for children or youth." To do otherwise, he insists, "is bordering on criminal behavior" (Horton, 1992, p. 11). In both his views and his language, he greatly resembles Mary Hunt. He further asserts that:

It is patent nonsense to suggest teaching the responsible use of an illegal substance. After all, drinking alcoholic beverages is illegal for adolescents in all states. If one accepts this approach, it would make just as much sense to teach the responsible use of cocaine or heroin." (Horton, 1992, p. 8)

His position seems remarkably similar to that of the early temperance activist Lyman Beecher, who preached that "much is said about the prudent use of spirits, but we might as well speak of the prudent use of the plague of fire handled prudently round among powder—of poison taken prudently every day" (Furnas, 1965, p. 65).

The unqualified blanket assertion that alcohol is illegal for young people is clearly incorrect. Those who are under the age of 21 can use alcohol, for example, in religious ceremonies and at home under the supervision of parents or guardians. But reduction-of-consumption advocates typically gloss over such matters (Chapman, 1991, p. 382), sometimes with a vengeance: "Carter Loar, a senior at Park View High School in Loudoun County, Virginia was suspended for ten days in February for violating the schools' alcohol policy" (*Campus Report*, 1995, p. 2). Carter's violation was using mouthwash at school. School officials confiscated the contraband and "He was charged with violating the school's alcohol policy which prohibits the possession or use of alcohol on school property. As part of his ten day suspension, Carter was required to attend a three day Substance Abuse Program sponsored by Loudoun County" (*Campus Report*, 1995, p. 2). One can only shudder to imagine what severe punishment he would have suffered had his crime been taking medication such as Comtrex (20% alcohol), Nyquil Cough Syrup (25% alcohol), or tincture of belladonna (67% alcohol) (Anderson, 1989, p. 69).

More importantly, the belief that teaching young people a sociocultural approach to alcohol is self-defeating, dangerous, or illegal is itself erroneous and illogical. Teaching about responsible use does not involve student consumption of alcohol any more than teaching them world geography involves their visiting Nepal, or teaching them civics involves their running for governor or voting for president. Such "programs would not encourage underage drinking, but would acknowledge the reality of alcohol experimentation. They would encourage thoughtful decisions and responsible behavior, incorporating information about drinking that an individual could use as an adult" (Engs and Fors, 1988, p. 27). Stated differently, "minors will soon be of legal drinking age, and should know how to be responsible drinkers before that time" (General Accounting Office, 1991, p. 62). On the basis of their study, Forney and his colleagues (1988, p. 194) concluded that "efforts to educate youth about alcohol should incorporate acceptable uses as well as the negative aspects of drinking." They explained that:

Promoting responsible attitudes by alcohol-education efforts, we believe, should include information concerning the acceptable uses of alcohol. Emphasis on the unacceptable uses of alcohol alone does not appear to deter students from drinking. This finding is supported by our study showing that over half of our students in grades six through twelve are currently drinking, 18% of them frequently or heavily. We believe that efforts to curb frequent or heavy drinking among adolescents must focus on promoting responsible drinking behaviors and attitudes.
    Alcohol is part of our society and it seems clear that most adolescents will experiment with it. Leaving students to find out about alcohol on their own may lead to serious consequences. Effective sources of information should help students decide when and how alcohol use is acceptable. (Forney et al., 1988, pp. 201–202)

As health educators St. Pierre and Miller (1986, p. 11) emphasized, "Alcohol education can provide the skills for adolescents and adults to abstain or to include alcohol as a part of the social situation. Through proper education, alcohol can be incorporated into the lifestyles of post-adolescent adults and older members of society without the traditional problems which [sometimes] accompany drinking in a social setting." Similarly, Carl May observed that:

socialization about alcohol *use* is experienced almost entirely outside of the school. In the current climate, at least, it is not politically possible for school-based packages to stress 'harm reduction' as a desirable objective, although that may be precisely what the practical business of learning to drink is about. In this context, it is impossible not to echo O'Connor and Saunders' (1992, p. 180) argument that: "if educational activity is to persist then we will probably be better served by training our young people to drink safely." Given this, the question of where and how such education be delivered is important. A potential way of achieving this is by building on the existing educational efforts of parents. (May, 1993, p. 163, emphasis in original)

As Chng pointed out:

The goal of abstinence implies that the school not only has primary responsibility for influencing behavior, but has full capacity for changing behavior as well. On the contrary, it is important to remember that much education does occur outside the school. The school is only one among many influences on the attitudes and behavior of the individual. Consequently, abstinence is an unrealistic, impractical goal because non-school influences sometimes may either nullify the effect of the school or render it unnecessary. The media, the peer group, and the family inevitably transmit their own form of "drug education" regardless of the intentions of the school. . . . It seems clear that drug education has not, and never will be able to accomplish this goal of abstinence. If it persists in retaining and promoting this goal, the cost of this "failure" may be severe. (Chng, 1981, pp. 16–17)

Even religious groups theologically committed to abstinence are not highly successful in maintaining it among their members. For example, the Seventh-Day Adventist Church lists the "use, manufacture, or sale of alcoholic beverages" as grounds for expulsion from the church, it publishes two periodicals promoting abstinence among both elementary and high school students and it operates an extensive system of schools and colleges "in order to provide an education in harmony with Adventist belief from kindergarten through graduate school" (Guthrie, 1986, pp. 8, 11). Yet in spite of the religious basis for abstinence, reinforced through education and strong social pressure, nearly sixty percent of seniors enrolled in a sample of Seventh-Day Adventist academies reported drinking (Guthrie, 1986, p. 79). The same is true for the Church of Jesus Christ of Latter-day Saints ("Mormon" Church) and other religious groups that require and attempt to enforce abstinence (Hanson, 1995, pp. 45–50). Why should we expect secular alcohol education to even reach this low level of success?

There is absolutely no reason, based on either theory or empirical research, to expect a no-use approach to be any more effective in alcohol education than it has been in other areas, such as human sexuality (Engs and Fors, 1988, p. 26). The strict no-use approach was not effective in Mary Hunt's day and it is not effective today.

Most college students drink and most of them, contrary to the common stereotype, typically drink in moderation. However, collegians drink within a set of norms differing from those in the larger society. Furthermore, often being away from home for the first time, they may experiment with excessive drinking behavior as part of normal development. During the freshman year, in particular, they may test the limits by staying up late, sleeping late, eating too much of the wrong foods, and similar excessive behavior. Haines (1983, p. 3) observed that "It is precisely for these reasons that college students are an ideal population at an opportune stage of development to be taught healthy drinking practices. As early as 1976 *The Whole College Catalog About Drinking* listed '. . . communicate what constitutes safe drinking practices for those who choose to drink' among its four fundamental goals of alcohol abuse prevention (DHEW, 1976)" (Haines, 1983, p. 3).[1]

A narrow-minded insistence on abstinence as the only option will cause students to "turn off and tune out" of alcohol education (Spowart, 1982, pp. 3–4). "It is at odds with the prevailing norms of adult behavior" and it "diverts attention away from what is probably achievable to what is almost an impossibility" (O'Connor and Saunders, 1992, pp. 167–168). Furthermore, "there is little value in perpetuating a perspective that emphasizes *don't* but persuades few not to while simultaneously ignoring those who do" (O'Connor and Saunders, 1992, p. 178, emphasis in original).

Long ago, Robinson noted that most alcohol education focused on the dire results and tragic consequences that could occur from alcohol misuse and made them appear almost inevitable. He stressed that:

We have often failed to recognize the fact that the majority of young people who choose to drink do not end up dead, or in hospital, in jail, or pregnant. We usually fail to acknowledge that there are distinct pleasures and real benefits in drinking alcoholic beverages in an appropriate and non-damaging way. This one-sided, negative kind of teaching, which runs contrary to the experience of a great many young people as well as the experience of a majority of older social drinkers, substantially reduces the believability of all our teaching. Unless our teaching materials and our handling of this topic in the classroom present fairer statements of fact, balanced realistically between the rewards and punishments that do occur in the experience of alcoholic beverage users, the effectiveness of teaching on this topic cannot be increased. (Robinson, 1969, p. 3)

The General Accounting Office (GAO) examined the policies and methods used by the Department of Education and the Department of Health and Human Services (HHS) in their efforts to identify and publicly recognize exemplary drug abuse prevention programs. It reported that:

The policies underlying both recognition efforts limited eligible programs to those with a "no-use" approach to drug abuse prevention for youths. In the strictest sense, no-use programs are those with a consistent message that any use of drugs, alcohol, or tobacco is always wrong and harmful. Responsible-use approaches, on the other hand, while *not* condoning the use of drugs, alcohol, or tobacco, may attempt to prevent or delay the onset of substance use by stressing informed decision making, or may aim to reduce the riskiest forms of use (such as drinking and driving) and encourage reduction in use *for those who are already involved* in tobacco, alcohol, and drug use. Current research evidence has not demonstrated the general superiority of one prevention approach over any other, nor have any evaluations isolated the effects of a no-use approach. Further, responsible-use approaches are widespread, as shown by the continued presence of Students Against Driving Drunk (SADD) chapters in 25,000 middle and high schools. (GAO, 1991, p. 2, emphasis in original)

Authors of the report explained that they:

found evidence of pessimism concerning the strict adherence to a no-use philosophy, despite the belief by many that this is the only sound approach. Polich et al. (1984) noted that because of the wide use and acceptability of alcohol, no existing approaches (including no use) would likely be successful against adolescent drinking. Moskowitz (1989) showed evidence of a lack of consensus about whether abstinence or responsible use is the most [sic] appropriate goal with regard to the use of alcohol. Goodstadt (1988) also noted that a no-use approach ignores the realities of use and further that more responsible use of a substance may be an appropriate intermediate goal of a program aimed at populations who use them. (GAO, 1991, p. 51)

The authors concluded that "there is no empirical evidence showing that one approach is more successful than another, and likewise there is no evidence that either would encourage alcohol or drug use (GAO, 1991, p. 51). They observed that "In the long run, if unproven programs receive recognition and later evidence shows that they are ineffective, two unfortunate consequences can follow: (1) all the other programs recognized may also be tarnished, and (2) public funds will have been wasted on any replication of the ineffective programs" (GAO, 1991, p. 45), to which might be added that (3) time will have been wasted pursuing false leads. The chance of this occurring are very high given the incredible fact that neither the Department of Education nor HHS requires any *evidence* whatsoever of effectiveness to designate a program as exemplary (GAO, 1991, p. 3). What *is* required is that all such programs pass the test of no-use purity. Mary Hunt would have been most pleased.

The GAO recommended that the two federal agencies *not* exclude responsible-use approaches from consideration of effectiveness, a recommendation that they both have adamantly rejected (GAO, 1991, p. 5). It is clear that *ideology rather than science prevails.*

OPPONENTS OF RESPONSIBLE DRINKING ARE MISGUIDED

In attempting to justify their opposition, opponents of the responsible drinking approach often reveal their misconceptions. For example, Chassey and Clifford (1988, pp. 275–276) incorrectly assert that:

1. The concept assumes that everyone drinks.
2. It puts a premium on drinking as "proof" of responsibility.
3. It assumes that everyone should drink, and allows no freedom for those who choose not to drink.

It is difficult to understand how anyone could be so completely incorrect about an approach that presents abstinence as an equally acceptable and desirable choice. Similarly, Chapman (1991, p. 382) identifies what he considers to be inherent flaws to promoting responsible drinking. "At best, the definition of responsible drinking is often arbitrary and capricious, given in an attempt to impress faculty or administrators while addressing a fear of alienating the student." This assertion implicitly recognizes that the definition of responsible drinking is *not* necessarily or usually arbitrary and capricious; the judgement of motive appears to be irrelevant. He also asserts that "Those who do not drink responsibly, by definition, drink irresponsibly. This is a judgmental characterization that tends to moralize about the compulsive drinking done by the individual with alcoholism." Of course, for alcoholics, responsible drinking is the consumption of non-alcoholic beverages. Those who drink irresponsibly must be criticized strongly for doing so. He also contends that "For those with alcoholism, try as they will, they cannot drink 'responsibly.'" Again, for alcoholics, the responsible choice is drinking non-alcoholic beverages. Chapman finally contends that "The term *responsible drinking* implies the consumption of some alcohol when there may well be individuals predisposed (genetically or environmentally) to alcohol abuse and alcoholism, thus at risk with *any* consumption of alcohol" (emphasis in original). At the risk of repetition, it must be pointed out yet again that advocates of the responsible drinking approach stress that for such individuals drinking non-alcoholic beverages is the responsible choice. Such opponents ignore the frequently stated objectives of responsible-use programs:

1. *Teach those who choose to drink to do so responsibly.* Help them learn to use alcohol in a way that is not detrimental to anyone.
2. *Reinforce those who choose not to drink.* Help them to resist peer pressure and create activities that are not alcohol related. (Upcraft and Eck, 1986, p. 37, emphases in original)

CONFUSION EXISTS

Apparently in response to Department of Education assertions, some states have indicated their unwillingness to use alcohol education materials that present a responsible use message rather than a strict no-use message, based on their belief that this is unacceptable under the Drug-Free Schools and Communities Act and might jeopardize both funding under that act and other federal programs. However, the Drug-Free Schools and Communities Act does not mandate a strict no-use message, irrespective of the desires of the Department of Education (Title V, Sec. 5144 [Materials]).

OBJECTIVITY AND OPEN-MINDEDNESS NEEDED

The evidence presented in the preceding chapter suggests that a responsible-use approach might well be more effective than a no-use approach in reducing alcohol problems. The GAO (1991, p. 37) stressed that:

While there is not a consensus about the merits of no-use versus responsible-use approaches, there is also no empirical evidence of the harmfulness or superiority of either approach. In the absence of such evidence and the presence of widespread drug use in our nation, the goals of the recognition effort would therefore be best met by allowing consideration of a wide range of approaches and by awarding recognition on the basis of merit and evidence of effectiveness. In this way, if either approach was found to be not generally effective in preventing drug use, the search for effective models would not have to begin anew.

Therefore, *we must promote the development and assessment of diverse curricula based on a sociocultural understanding of how best to reduce alcohol abuse.* Given the dismal record of no-use curricula, it would be negligent and irresponsible not to pursue a more promising approach. Additionally, we must take positive action to make up for the valuable time lost by governmental stonewalling of open research and investigation. For this reason *we must demand that federal agencies give priority to research on responsible drinking educational approaches for a period of at least 10 years.*

At a personal level, we don't need to wait for a change in governmental policy. We can emulate the good example of those groups that successfully enjoy alcohol with virtually no problems. *If we use alcohol responsibly and expect our children to enjoy it responsibly as adults, then we need to teach this to our children from an early age.* Our good example will be the most powerful education possible. By both word and deed (but most importantly by deed) we need to teach them that alcohol is a natural and normal part of life; that it is neither poison nor elixir; that drinking in moderation and abstaining are equally desirable choices; and that the abuse of alcohol is always totally and completely unacceptable. By letting them enjoy alcohol beverages within the home under our supervision, they learn moderation and responsible consumption and also realize that the consumption of alcohol is not a sign of adulthood. Teaching our children to drink in moderation, if they choose to drink, is not a radical idea, but one that was practiced by our earliest European settlers and the founders of our republic.

The GAO (1991, pp. 3–4) also found a tendency by the Department of Education to favor certain teaching techniques (such as resistance skills training and self-esteem enhancement) over others (such as peer programs and alternatives approaches) that show much promise in the research literature. Such bias can be counterproductive and is not in the best interest of students. Accordingly, *we must promote the vigorous and open-minded exploration of the effectiveness of a diversity of teaching strategies.* Anything short of this would be an unethical abrogation of responsibility and would short-change our youth.

SCARE TACTICS ARE COMMON

While scare tactics have largely been discredited in alcohol education, they can effectively be used to convince the public of the need to take action. For example, an investigator reported that as many as 90 percent of the students at one Eastern university drank in their freshman year, 95 percent drank in their senior year, 35 percent drank heavily, and 15 percent became alcoholics. The year of the study was 1903! While one should obviously question the objectivity of the writer and the accuracy of these apparently inflated statistics because they were based on observations, talking with faculty and students, and "examination of records" and that they were reported in a book titled *The Demoralization of College Life* (Crane, 1911, p. 14), the author was probably successful in influencing public opinion.

Unfortunately, shoddy and deceptive research did not end at the turn of the century. The use of inflated, distorted, and even fabricated statistics is a serious problem today, polluting and misleading the discussion of public issues. A report recently asserted that the proportion of college women who drank to become intoxicated had increased over threefold between 1977 and 1993 and asserted ominously that binge drinking had reached epidemic proportions, the disastrous consequences of which posed a major threat to the very life of America's most precious asset, its young people (Center on Addiction and Substance Abuse, 1994, p. ii). The authors reported that 90 percent of all campus rapes occur when alcohol is being used and that 60 percent of college women who have contracted sexually transmitted diseases such as AIDS were under the influence of alcohol at the time of infection. Major newspapers across the country carried the story as front page news with such headlines as "College Binge Drinking Soars" and "College Students of America Wade Deeper Into Sea of Booze." It was featured on network evening news stories and reported in news magazines and newspaper columns. Reporters should have questioned the credibility of the report given the fact that it was based entirely on such apparently flimsy research as "interviews, focus groups, hearings, and reviews of available data and literature" (Center on Addiction and Substance Abuse at Columbia University, 1994, p. 1) and was funded by a neo-dry foundation.

The report's assertion that 90 percent of all reported campus rapes occur when alcohol is being used was a statistic not supported by any footnote, a statistic that does not appear to exist in the published research on rape, and a statistic that was not supported by any original research by the authors. The Center on Addiction and Substance Abuse at Columbia University (CASA) was subsequently unable to provide any support whatsoever for this sensational assertion, which appears to have been pulled from thin air (McNamara-Meis, 1995, p. 22). Similarly, the assertion that 60 percent of college women who have contracted sexually transmitted diseases such as AIDS were under the influence of alcohol is also totally speculative and without any foundation in fact.

The assertion that there had been a threefold increase in the proportion of college women drinking to get drunk between 1977 and 1993 was not only totally unsupported but highly inconsistent with all the research conducted over that time period by researchers, none of whom were apparently contacted by reporters (McNamara-Meis, 1995, p. 21).

Even the most improbable of statistics are repeated by news media as fact and become part of public belief. For example, it is now widely believed by the public that the average 18 year old has seen 100,000 beer commercials on television. The origin of this statistic was "Myths, Men & Beer," a lengthy report on beer commercials that appeared on network television in 1987. The report, written by four college faculty members, was paid for and published by a private organization. It was not reviewed by academic peers and was never published in a scholarly journal. While data from A.C. Neilsen Company and the Aribtron Company demonstrate the falsity of the 100,000 beer commercial claim, common sense alone should be enough to dispel the myth. Sixteen years or about 5,844 days occur between a person's second and eighteenth birthday. To see 100,000 beer commercials in that time, a person would have to see an average of more than seventeen a day! But this clearly absurd statistic was gullibly repeated over and over:

- "According to Neil Postman, professor of media ecology at New York University, and his colleagues, children see more than 100,000 beer commercials before they are old enough to legally drink and drive."—From a bylined article by Patricia Taylor, director of the Alcohol Policies Project of the Center for Science in the Public Interest, in the *New York Times*, March 20, 1988.
- "Four academicians under the auspices of the AAA Foundation for Traffic Safety recently . . . analyzed the content of 40 such (beer) commercials broadcast on network television during February and March 1987. Their major concern was the effect of these messages on children, because as the report says, 'between the ages of 2 and 18,

the period in which social learning is most intense, American children see something like 100,000 television commercials for beer.'"—*Sports Illustrated*, Aug. 1, 1988.

- "Alcohol marketing and advertising provides the single greatest source of alcohol education for American children. Our children will see close to 100,000 television commercials for beer alone by the time they are 18."—Testimony in support of warning labels on alcoholic beverage containers to the Senate Subcommittee on Consumer Affairs (Sen. Albert Gore, Jr., chairman) by Christine Lupinski, Washington representative for the National Council on Alcoholism on behalf of Coalition for Health and Safety Warnings on Alcoholic Beverages, Aug. 10, 1988.

- "American children see an estimated 100,000 beer ads on television before they are old enough to legally drink and drive." —From a letter in support of warning labels by J. Scott Douglas, director, The Committee For Children, submitted as part of the Gore subcommittee hearing record, Aug. 10, 1988.

- "I read an article in a paper yesterday stating that children from 2 to 18 years old see at least 100,000 advertisements a year (*sic*) concerning alcohol in some form."—From a statement in support of warning labels, offered at the same hearing by Senator Strom Thurmond of South Carolina.

- "A two-year-old child growing up in America will see about 100,000 beer commercials by the time he or she is 18. But that will change if U.S. Surgeon General C. Everett Koop and a vocal group of consumer and public health activists have their way."—Lead of story in *San Francisco Examiner*, Feb. 19, 1989.

- "They will see 100,000 (beer) commercials by the time they turn 18."—Jean Kilbourne, member of the National Council on Alcoholism, as quoted in the *Austin American Statesman*, Oct. 15, 1989.

- "I think the industry is flooding the nation with these not so subtle messages to drink on every possible occasion, so the occasional message of knowing when to say when interspersed with 100,000 other messages that go out, that young people have seen by the time they're 21, really isn't doing much good. . . ."—Doris Aiken, president of Remove Intoxicated Drivers (RID), speaking on "Sonya Live in L.A.," a Cable Network News Broadcast, Dec. 5, 1989.

- "The fact that kids can see as many as 100,000 beer commercials before they're of legal drinking age really sets a tone about alcohol that really needs to be changed."—Patricia Taylor, director of the Alcohol Policies Project of the Center for Science in the Public Interest, in an interview on Consumer News Business Channel, Dec. 22, 1989.

- "Children, he (Dr. Koop) said, see 100,000 beer commercials by the time they turn 18."—Statement attributed to former Surgeon General C. Everett Koop, from an article in the *New York Times*, Feb. 14, 1990 (Anheuser-Busch Companies, n.d., addendum).

This blatantly absurd statistic has even found its way into textbooks for students and in materials for teachers (Baker, 1993, p. 215; Horton, 1992, p. 23).

Distorted, biased, or incorrect statistics may attract media attention. They may even influence public policy. But they cannot contribute to a reduction of alcohol abuse, which requires accurate information and unbiased interpretation. Therefore, *we must be skeptical of surprising, sensationalized statistics*. Typically, the inflated statistics will be associated with talk of epidemics, threats to our youth, and similar alarmist language. Often the statistics will be promoted by groups with laudable sounding names such as the Center for Science in the Public Interest, which some regard as a political advocacy group rather than an objective scientific organization. Groups such as the Center for Science in the Public Interest, which may have an underlying political agenda, often tend to exaggerate the extent and growth of problems in which they have an interest and, typically, a proposed solution. Problems widely seen by the public as being of epidemic proportion justify ever larger budgets, increased staffs, higher salaries, more power, and greater organizational prestige. Such groups clearly have a vested interest in exaggeration. We must maintain a stronger public interest in insisting on accuracy and on not being deceived and stampeded into simplistic solutions to complex problems.

Reporters have an important role in demanding accuracy. Because they cannot be experts on everything, they must not only ask critical questions in general, but must ascertain the credibility of the research on which press releases are based. Unfortunately, research techniques are ordinarily so technical that most journalists, especially under the pressure of time, will necessarily need to rely on the judgment of experts. For this reason, *reporters must routinely ask if the research in question has been accepted by a peer-reviewed publication and, if not, they must ask if it has been submitted for evaluation to the Statistical Assessment Service.*[2] If neither has been done; reporters should ask why it has not, should be especially skeptical, and should ask why they should not ignore the research. *The burden of proof must be shifted to those who present research to demonstrate its credibility.* That is the nature of science; it is definitely not the practice of self-aggrandizing advocacy groups that would deceive us. Reporters and the public have been misled too often and the public interest requires that it be stopped.

CONCLUSION

Alcohol has been used around the world for thousands of years. Some societies and groups widely and extensively consume beverage alcohol with very few problems while others experience much misuse. By analyzing those who use it successfully, we can apply their techniques in our own use of alcohol. Italians, Greeks, Jews, and others tend to share three common keys to success:

- First, there is an absence of emotionality associated with alcohol, which is seen as a natural and normal part of life. It is seen as neither a poison on the one hand, nor as a solution to life's problems on the other.
- Second, there is little or no social pressure to drink. Abstaining and drinking in moderation as seen as equally desirable or acceptable choices. However, the abuse of alcohol is never tolerated for any reason.
- Third, young people learn at home from their parents and their parents' good example how to handle alcohol responsibly.

Neo-prohibitionists reject human experience and insist that we must further restrict the availability of alcohol. This is because:

They assume that reducing alcohol availability reduces total alcohol consumption, which reduces heavy drinker prevalence, which reduces drunkenness and related problems. Hence, it is claimed that the government can prevent alcohol problems by controlling the first cause in this linear causal chain—alcohol availability. To the extent that this shift in the source of drunkenness from the drinker back to alcohol becomes popular, Americans will have come full circle back to the alcohol mythology that spawned the ill-fated Prohibition experiment. (Mulford, 1994, p. 518)

We need to accept the wisdom of the ancient Chinese proverb: intoxication is not the fault of the alcohol but of the person (Billings, 1905, pp. 40–41).[3]

NOTES

1. It was shortly after this time (mid-1977) that federal policy began moving toward the reduction-of-consumption approach (Parker, 1984; Blocker, 1989).

2. The Statistical Assessment Service, a non-profit organization, is located in Suite 300 at 2100 L. Street, N.W. in Washington, D.C. 20037. (202) 223–3194.

3. Billings (1905, p. 41) used the more traditional translation, "Intoxication is not the wine's fault, but the man's."

References

Aaron, Paul, and Musto, David. Temperance and Prohibition in America: An Historical Overview. In: Moore, Mark H., and Gerstein, Dean R. (eds.) *Alcohol and Public Policy: Beyond the Shadow of Prohibition.* Washington, DC: National Academy Press, 1981. pp. 127–181.

Alaska Council on Prevention of Alcohol and Drug Abuse, Inc. *Evaluation of the Statewide Alcohol Education Project, "Here's Looking at You, Two" Alcohol Education Curriculum.* Anchorage, AK: Alaska Council on Prevention of Alcohol and Drug Abuse, Inc., 1982.

Allison, Kenneth R., Silverman, Gloria, and Dignam, Carol. Effects on students of teacher training in use of a drug education curriculum. *Journal of Drug Education,* 1990, *20,* 31–46.

American Council on Alcohol Problems. *Introducing—American Council on Alcohol Problems.* Bridgeton, MO: American Council on Alcohol Problems, n.d.

American Library Association. *The National Union Catalog: Pre-1956 Imprints.* London, England: Mansell. 1973.

Ametrano, Irene M. An evaluation of the effectiveness of a substance-abuse prevention program. *Journal of College Student Development,* 1992, *33,* 507–515.

Anderson, David. The Meaning of Alcoholism. Presentation to College of Education faculty, Michigan State University, 1979.

Anderson, David (ed.). *A Winning Combination: An Alcohol, Other Drug, and Traffic Safety Handbook for College Campuses.* Washington, DC: National Highway Traffic Safety Administration, 1989.

Andrews, M. The knowledge, attitudes, and behavior concerning alcohol use of resident assistants and residence hall students. *Journal of Alcohol and Drug Education,* 1987, *33,* 86–90.

Andrews, Richard L., and Hearne, Jill T. Effects of primary grades health curriculum project on student and parent smoking attitudes and behavior. *Journal of School Health,* 1984, *54,* 18–20.

Anheuser-Busch Companies. *100,000 Beer Commercials?* St. Louis, MO: Anheuser-Busch Companies, n.d.

Anti-Saloon League of America. *Anti-Saloon League of America Yearbook.* Westerville, OH: American Issue Press, 1920, p. 28. Cited by Mulford, Harold A. *Alcohol and Alcoholism in Iowa, 1965.* Iowa City, IA: University of Iowa, 1965, p. 9.

Archibald, Norman. College Administrator and Student Perceptions Relative to Probable Effectiveness of Alcohol Education Programs. Unpublished Ed.D. dissertation, Texas Tech University, 1985.

Argentos, Mary J. The Evaluation of a Drug and Alcohol Prevention Program in a Secondary School Setting. Unpublished Ph.D. dissertation, University of Oklahoma, 1991.

Arndt, Anthony L. The Relationship between Knowledge of Alcohol and Change in Attitudes and Behavior Toward Alcohol in an Alcohol Education Program. Unpublished M.S. thesis, University of Wisconsin at Stout, 1979.

Asbury, Herbert. *The Great Illusion: An Informal History of Prohibition.* New York: Greenwood Press, 1968 (Originally published 1950).

Bacon, Selden D. Meeting the Problem of Alcoholism in the United States. In: Whitney, Elizabeth D. (ed.) *World Dialogue on Alcohol and Drug Dependence.* Boston, MA: Beacon Press, 1970. pp. 134–145.

Bader, Robert S. *Prohibition in Kansas: A History.* Lawrence, KS: University Press of Kansas, 1986.

Baer, John S., Kivlahan, Daniel R., Fromme, Kim, and Marlatt, G. Alan. Secondary Prevention of Alcohol Abuse with College Student Populations: A Skills-Training Approach. In: Howard, George S., and Nathan, Peter E. (eds.) *Alcohol Use and Misuse by Young Adults.* Notre Dame, IN: University of Notre Dame Press, 1994. pp. 83–108.

Baer, Paul E., McLaughlin, Robert J., Burnside, Mary A., and Pokorny, Alex D. Alcohol use and psychosocial outcome of two preventive classroom programs with seventh and tenth graders. *Journal of Drug Education,* 1988, *18,* 171–184.

Bagnall, Gellisse, and Plant, Martin A. Education on drugs and alcohol: Past disappointments and future challenges. *Health Education Research,* 1987, *2,* 417–422.

Baker, Falcon. Toward a Winnable War on Drugs. In: Goldberg, Raymond (ed.) *Taking Sides: Clashing Views on Controversial Issues in Drugs and Society.* Guilford, CT: Dushkin Publishing, 1993. pp. 212–216.

Baldy, Marian W. *The University Wine Course: A Wine Appreciation Text and Self Tutorial.* San Francisco, CA: Wine Appreciation Guild, 1993.

Barnett, Milton L. Alcoholism in the Cantonese of New York City: An Anthropological Study. In: Diethelm, Oskar (ed.) *Etiology of Chronic Alcoholism.* Springfield, IL: Charles C. Thomas, 1955. pp. 179–227.

Beam, III, Augustus P. Alcohol-Related Knowledge, Attitudes, and Behavior of College Undergraduates. Unpublished M.S. thesis, North Carolina State University at Raleigh, 1981.

Beauchamp, Dan E. Alcohol-Abuse Prevention Through Beverage and Environmental Regulation: Where We Have Been and Where We Are Going. In: Holder, Harold D. (ed.) *Advances in Substance Abuse: Behavioral and Biological Research* Supplement 1. Greenwich, CT: JAI Press, 1987. pp. 53–63.

Becker, Harold K., Agopian, Michael W., and Yeh, Sandy. Impact evaluation of Drug Abuse Resistance Education (DARE). *Journal of Drug Education.* 1992, *22,* 283–291.

Bell, Robert M., Ellickson, Phyllis L., and Harrison, Ellen R. Do drug prevention effects persist into high school? How Project ALERT did with ninth graders. *Preventive Medicine,* 1993, *22,* 463–483.

Benard, Bonnie. Characteristics of effective prevention programs. *Prevention Forum,* 1986, *6,* 3–8.

Billings, John S. *Physiological Aspects of the Liquor Problem: Investigations Made by and Under the Direction of U. O. Atwater, John S. Billings and Others. Sub-Committee of the Committee of Fifty to Investigate the Liquor Problem.* Boston: Houghton, Mifflin, 1903.

Billings, John S. (ed.). *The Liquor Problem: A Summary of Investigations Conducted by the Committee of Fifty, 1893–1903.* Boston: Houghton, Mifflin, 1905.

Blacker, Edward. Sociocultural factors in alcoholism. *International Psychiatry Clinics,* 1966, *3*, 51–80.

Blane, Howard T. Education and the Prevention of Alcoholism. In: Kissin, Benjamin, and Begleiter, Henri (eds.) *Social Aspects of Alcoholism: The Biology of Alcoholism* New York, NY: Plenum Press, 1978. pp. 519–578.

Blocker, Jr., Jack S. *Retreat from Reform.* Westport, CT: Greenwood Press, 1976.

Blocker, Jr., Jack S. *"Give to the Winds thy Fear": The Women's Temperance Crusade, 1873–1874.* Westport, CT: Greenwood Press, 1985.

Blocker, Jr., Jack S. *American Temperance Movements: Cycles of Reform.* Boston, MA: Twayne, 1989.

Blom, Gaston E., and Snoddy, James E. The Child, the Teacher, and the Drinking Society: A Conceptual Framework for Alcohol Education in the Elementary School. In: Mayer, John E., and Filstead, William J. (eds.) *Adolescence and Alcohol.* Cambridge, MA: Ballinger, 1980. pp. 257–272.

Blum, Steven B., Rivers, Clayton, Horvat, Joseph, and Bellows, David. The effect of contracted abstinence on college students' behavior toward alcohol use. *Journal of Alcohol and Drug Education,* 1980, *25*, 70–77.

Bonaguro, John A., Rhonehouse, Michael, and Bonaguro, Ellen W. Effectiveness of four school health education projects upon substance use, self-esteem, and adolescent stress. *Health Education Quarterly,* 1988, *15*, 81–92.

Bonilla, Doris S. Preventive Alcohol Education: Effect on Middle School Students' Attitude Toward Alcohol. Unpublished M.S. thesis, University of South Carolina, 1993.

Bordin, Ruth. *Woman and Temperance: The Quest for Power and Liberty, 1873–1900.* Philadelphia, PA: Temple University Press, 1981.

Botvin, Gilbert J. *Life Skills Training: Teacher's Manual.* New York: Smithfield Press, 1981.

Botvin, Gilbert J., Baker, Eli, Botvin, Elizabeth M., Filazzola, Anne D., and Milman, Robert B. Prevention of alcohol misuse through the development of personal and social competence: A pilot study. *Journal of Studies on Alcohol,* 1984a, *45*, 550–552.

Botvin, Gilbert J., Baker, Eli, Dusenbury, Linda, Tortu, Stephanie, and Botvin, Elizabeth M. Preventing adolescent drug abuse through a multimodel cognitive-behavioral approach: Results of a 3-year study. *Journal of Consulting and Clinical Psychology,* 1990, *58*, 437–446.

Botvin, Gilbert J., Baker, Eli, Renick, Nancy L., Filazzola, Anne D., and Botvin, Elizabeth M. A cognitive-behavioral approach to substance abuse prevention. *Addictive Behaviors,* 1984b, *9*, 137–147.

Botvin, Gilbert J., Renick, Nancy L., and Baker, Eli. The effects of scheduling format and booster sessions on a broad-spectrum psychosocial smoking prevention program. *Journal of Behavioral Medicine,* 1983, *6*, 359–379.

Bowling, John B. Effects of a Minimal Cognitive Intervention on the Alcohol-Related Knowledge and Attitudes of Fraternity Members. Unpublished M.S. thesis, University of Maine, 1991.

Bradley, Dianne F. Alcohol and drug education in the elementary school. *Elementary School Guidance and Counseling,* 1988, *23*, 99–105.

Bremberg, Sven, and Arborelius, Elizabeth. Effects on adolescent alcohol consumption of a school based student-centered health counselling programme. *Scandinavian Journal of Social Medicine*, 1994, *22*, 113–119.

Brooks, Vicki S. Alcohol Education Pedagogy: Effects on Knowledge and Locus of Control. Unpublished Ph.D. dissertation, University of Wyoming, 1992.

Brown, Deborah E. A Study of Knowledge Gain by At-Risk Middle School Students Participating in a Drug and Alcohol Education Program. Unpublished M.S.W. thesis, Rhode Island College, 1990.

Burch, Genevieve. *Alcohol Prevention in Five Secondary Schools: Effectiveness of an Education/Counseling/Advising Program*. Omaha, NE: University of Nebraska, Center for Applied Urban Research, 1980.

Burnham, John C. New perspectives on the prohibition "experiment" of the 1920's. *Journal of Social History*, 1968, *2*, 51–68.

Butler, J. Early adolescent alcohol consumption and self-concept, social class and knowledge of alcohol. *Journal of Studies on Alcohol*, 1982, *43*, 603–607.

Cahalan, Don. Why does the alcoholism field act like a ship of fools? *British Journal of Addiction*, 1979, *74*, 235–238.

Caleekal, John, Anuppa, and Pletsch, D. H. An interdisciplinary cognitive approach to alcohol education in the university curriculum. *Journal of Alcohol and Drug Education*, 1984, *30*, 50–60.

Camacho, Roberta A. The Effects of a Motion Picture Advance Organizer on the Learning of Information in Alcohol Education. Unpublished Ph.D. dissertation, Boston College, 1987.

Campanelli, Pamela C., Dielman, T. E., Shope, Jean T., Butchart, Amy T., and Renner, Deborah S. Pretest and treatment effects in an elementay school-based alcohol misuse prevention program. *Health Education Quarterly*, 1989, *16*, 113–130.

Campus Report. A pox on mouthwash. *Campus Report*, 1995 (April), *10*, 2.

Carl, Jacqueline J. A Comparison of the Effects of a Psychosocial Education Curriculum on Substance Knowledge, Attitude, Experience and Self-Esteem of High School Freshmen. Unpublished Ed.D. dissertation, University of Massachusetts, 1983.

Carpenter, Richard A. A Peer Managed Self-Control Program for Reduction of Alcohol Consumption in High School Students. Unpublished Ph.D. dissertation, Utah State University, 1981.

Cashman, Sean D. *Prohibition: The Lie of the Land*. New York: Free Press, 1981.

Casswell, Sally. The effect of pretesting on evaluation of a drug education program. *Journal of Drug Education*, 1982, *12*, 173–180.

Center on Addiction and Substance Abuse at Columbia University. *Rethinking Rites of Passage: Substance Abuse on America's Campuses—A Report by the Commission on Universities*. New York: Center on Addiction and Substance Abuse at Columbia University, June, 1994.

Chafetz, Morris E. Alcoholism prevention and reality. *Quarterly Journal of Studies on Alcohol*, 1967, *28*, 345–348.

Chafetz, Morris E. Problems of reaching youth. *Journal of School Health*, 1973, *43*, 40–44.

Chafetz, Morris E. Personal communication to Gaston E. Blom and James E. Snoddy, 1979.

Chapman, Robert J. Responsible drinking: A mistaken objective for collegiate alcohol programs. *Journal of College Student Development*, 1991, *32*, 381–382.

Chard-Yaron, Sharon D. The Effects of an Alcohol, Tobacco, and Other Drug Education/Prevention Curriculum on Selected Risk Factors for Substance Abuse. Unpublished Ed.D. dissertation, United States International University, 1992.

Chassey, Richard A., and Clifford, Deborah A. Responsibility versus choice: A different approach to alcohol education. *Journal of College Student Development*, 1988, *29*, 275–276.

Chen, William, and Bosch, Margaret. Comparison of drinking attitudes and behaviors between participating and non-participating students in a voluntary alcohol education program. *Journal of Alcohol and Drug Education*, 1987, *32*, 7–13.

Chen, W. William, Bosch, Margaret, and Cychosz, Charles M. The impact of a voluntary educational program—Tip It Lightly, Alcohol Awareness Week—on the drinking attitudes and behaviors of college students. *Journal of Drug Education*, 1982, *12*, 125–135.

Cherrington, Ernest H. *The Evolution of Prohibition in the United States of America.* Westerville, OH: American Issue Press, 1920.

Childs, Randolph W. *Making Repeal Work.* Philadelphia, PA: Pennsylvania Alcoholic Beverage Study, Inc., 1947.

Chng, Chwee L. A critique of values: Clarification in drug education. *Journal of Drug Education*, 1980, *10*, 119–125.

Chng, Chwee. L. The goal of abstinence: Implications for drug education. *Journal of Drug Education*, 1981, *11*, 13–18.

Cisin, Ira H. Formal and Informal Social Control over Drinking. In: Ewing, John A., and Rouse, Beatrice A. (eds.) *Drinking: Alcohol in American Society—Issues and Current Research.* Chicago, IL: Nelson-Hall, 1978. pp. 145–158.

Clark, Norman H. *The Dry Years: Prohibition and Social Change in Washington.* Seattle, WA: University of Washington Press, 1965.

Clark, N. H. *Deliver Us From Evil: An Interpretation of American Prohibition.* New York: Norton, 1976.

Claydon, Peter D. College Student Participation in Alcohol Education: Impact on Alcohol Knowledge, Attitudes and Behaviors. Unpublished Ph.D. dissertation, University of California at Santa Barbara, 1982.

Clayton, Richard R., Cattarello, Anne, Day, L. Edward, and Walden, Katherine P. Persuasive Communication and Drug Prevention: An Evaluation of the DARE Program. In: Donohew, Lewis, Sypher, Howard E., and Bukoski, William J. (eds.) *Persuasive Communication and Drug Abuse Prevention.* Hillsdale, NJ: Lawrence Erlbaum Associates, 1991. pp. 295–313.

Cleckler, Paula E. An Evaluation of An Educational Substance Abuse Prevention Program. Unpublished Ed.D. dissertation, University of Georgia, 1991.

Cohen, V. Study finds a little alcohol may lead to safer drinking. *Washington Post*, March 7, 1981, p. A-12.

Collins, Donna L. A Study of a Brief Alcohol Education Program. Unpublished M.S. thesis, Francis Marion College, 1990.

Collins, Donna, and Cellucci, Tony. Effects of a school-based alcohol education program with a media prevention component. *Psychological Reports*, 1991, *69*, 191–197.

Collins, Pamella C. The Long-Term and Short-Term Effects of an Alcohol Education Program Which Emphasizes Decision Making. Unpublished Ed.D. dissertion, East Texas State University, 1980.

Colvin, D. Leigh. *Prohibition in the United States: A History of the Prohibition Party and the Prohibition Movement.* New York: George H. Doran Co., 1926.

Conroy, D. W. Puritans and Tavern: Law and Popular Culture in Colonial Massachusetts, 1630–1720. Paper presented at the Conference on the Social History of Alcohol: Drinking and Culture and Modern Society. Berkeley, CA., 1984. Cited by Prendergast, Michael L. A History of Alcohol Problem Prevention Efforts in the United States. In:

Holder, Harold D. (ed.) *Control Issues in Alcohol Abuse Prevention: Strategies for States and Communities.* Greenwich, CT: JAI Press, 1987, p. 27.

Conyne, Robert K. Primary prevention through a campus alcohol education project. *Personnel and Guidance Journal* (Special issue: Primary Prevention on the Campus and in the Community), 1984, *62*, 524–528.

Cooper, Linda D. The Effectiveness of the Meeks-Heit Drug and Alcohol Education Curricular Unit on Sixth Graders' Attitude and Behavior Toward Alcohol Use. Unpublished M.S. thesis, University of Kansas, 1989.

Cowan, Richard. How the narcs created crack. *National Review*, 1986, *38*, pp. 26–28, 30–31.

Crane, Richard T. *The Demoralization of College Life.* Chicago, IL: H. O. Shepard Co., 1911.

DeJong, William. A short-term evaluation of Project DARE (Drug Abuse Resistance Education): Preliminary indications of effectiveness. *Journal of Drug Education*, 1987, *17*, 279–294.

DeLoughry, T. J. Colleges rush to comply with rules on fraud and drugs after Cavazos warns of aid cut-off. *The Chronicle of Higher Education*, 1989 (June 28), A1, A18.

DeLoughry, T. J. Bennett asks for an end to federal aid to colleges that fail to punish students for illegal drug use. *The Chronicle of Higher Education*, 1989b (August 16), A15, A20.

DeLoughry, T. J. President proposes to deny U.S. support to colleges that don't adopt "tough but fair" drug policies. *The Chronicle of Higher Education*, 1989c (September 13), A1, A30.

Demone, Jr., Harold W. The Nonuse and Abuse of Alcohol by the Male Adolescent. In: Chafetz, Morris E. (ed.) *Proceedings of the Second Annual Alcoholism Conference of the National Institute on Alcohol Abuse and Alcoholism.* Washington, DC: U.S. Government Printing Office, 1972.

Dennison, Darwin. A motivational model to modify actual health behavior. *Journal of School Health*, 1974, *44*, 16–20.

Dennison, Darwin. Activated health education. *Health Education*, 1977, *8*, 24–25.

Deutscher, Irwin. *What We Say/What We Do: Sentiments and Acts.* Glenview, IL: Scott, Foresman and Co., 1973.

DiCicco, Lena, Biron, Ronald, Carifo, James, Deutsch, Charles, Mills, Dixie J., Orenstein, Alan, Re, Andrea, Unterberger, Hilma, and White Robert E. Evaluation of the CASPAR alcohol education curriculum. *Journal of Studies on Alcohol*, 1984, *45*, 160–169.

DiCicco, Lena M., and Unterberger, Hilma. Cultural and professional avoidance: A dilemma in alcoholism training. *Journal of Alcohol and Drug Education*, 1977, *22*, 28–38.

Dielman, T. E., Kloska, Deborah D., Leech, Sharon L., Schulenberg, John E., and Shope, Jean T. Susceptibility to peer pressure as an explanatory variable for the differential effectiveness of an alcohol misuse prevention program in elementary schools. *Journal of School Health*, 1992, *62*, 233–237.

Dielman, T. E., Shope, Jean T., Butchart, Amy T., and Campanelli, Pamela C. Prevention of adolescent alcohol misuse: An elementary school program. *Journal of Pediatric Psychology*, 1986, *11*, 259–282.

Dielman, T. E., Shope, Jean T., Campanelli, Pamela C., and Butchart, Amy T. Elementary school-based prevention of adolescent alcohol misuse. *Pediatrician*, 1987, *14*, 70–76.

Dielman, T. E., Shope, Jean T., Leech, Sharon L., and Butchart, Amy T. Differential effectiveness of an elementary school-based alcohol misuse prevention program. *Journal of School Health*, 1989, *59*, 255–263.

Dignan, Mark B., Block, Geoffrey D., Steckler, Allan, and Cosby, Meredith. Evaluation of the North Carolina risk reduction program for smoking and alcohol. *Journal of School Health*, 1985, *55*, 103–106.

Dolan, J. S. Observations about the responsible drinking theme and THRESHOLD. *Journal of Alcohol and Drug Education*, 1976, *2*, 20–29.

Drug Free Schools and Campuses Rules, 34CFR86.100. Quoted by Palmer, Carolyn J., Gehring, Donald D., and Guthrie, Victoria L. Student knowledge of information mandated by the 1989 amendments to the Drug Free Schools and Communities Act. *NASPA Journal*, 1992, *30*, p. 31.

Dunn, Edward T. Health Knowledge, Health Teaching and Alcohol-Related Behavior. Unpublished Ed.D. dissertation, Boston University, 1981.

Dupont, Paul J., and Jason, Leonard A. Assertiveness training in a preventive drug education program. *Journal of Drug Education*, 1984, *14*, 369–378.

Durrell, Jack, and Bukoski, William. Primary Prevention of Drug Abuse: Major Promising Approaches. In: International Congress on Alcoholism and Drug Dependence. *Alcohol, Drugs and Tobacco: An International Perspective—Past, Present and Future: Proceedings of the 34th International Congress on Alcoholism and Drug Dependence, August 4–10, 1985, Calgary, Alberta, Canada.* Calgary: Alberta Alcohol and Drug Abuse Commission, 1985. pp. 377–379.

Duryea, Elias. Utilizing tenets of inoculation theory to develop and evaluate a preventive alcohol education intervention. *Journal of School Health*, 1983, *53*, 250–255.

Duryea, Elias. Student compliance in risky alcohol situations. *Journal of Alcohol and Drug Education*, 1985, *30*, 44–50.

Duryea, Elias, Mohr, Patricia, Newman, Ian M., Martin, Gary L., and Egwaoje, Emmanuel. Six-month follow-up results of a preventive alcohol education intervention. *Journal of Drug Education*, 1984, *14*, 97–104.

Duryea, Elias, and Okwumabua, Jebose O. Effects of a preventive alcohol education program after three years. *Journal of Drug Education*, 1988, *18*, 23–31.

Duston, Evelyn K., Kraft, David P., and Jaworski, Bernard. Alcohol education project: Preliminary answers. *Journal of the American College Health Association*, 1981, *29*, 272–278.

Eakin, Thomas J. An Evaluation Study of the Peer Education Component of the Total Alcohol Awareness Program (TAAP). Unpublished D.Ed. dissertation, Pennsylvania State University, 1984.

Education Commission of the States. Task Force on Responsible Decisions about Alcohol. *Final Report.* Denver, CO: Education Commission of the States. Task Force on Responsible Decisions about Alcohol. Booklet Number 2, n.d.

Egwaoje, Emmanuel S. Ninth Grade Preventive Alcohol Education: Six Months Later. Unpublished M.S. thesis, University of Nebraska, 1982.

Einstein, Stanley, Lavenhar, M., Wolfson, E., Louria, D., Quinones, M. and McAteer, G. The training of teachers for drug abuse education: Preliminary considerations. *Journal of Drug Education*, 1971, *1*, 323–345.

Ellickson, Phyllis, and Bell, Robert M. Drug prevention in junior high: A multi-site longitudinal test. *Science*, 1990, *247*, 1299–1305.

Ellickson, Phyllis L., Bell, Robert M., and Harrison, Ellen R. Changing adolescent propensities to use drugs: Results from project ALERT. *Health Education Quarterly*, 1993, *20*, 227–242.

Elwood, Kristina. The Effectiveness of the Drug Abuse Resistance Education Curricular Unit on Sixth Graders' Knowledge, Attitudes, and Behavior Toward Alcohol Use. Unpublished M.S. thesis, University of Kansas, 1991.

Emerson, Haven. Prohibition and morality and morbidity. *Annals of the American Academy of Political and Social Science*, 1932, *163*, 53–60.

E. M. J. (Presumably E. M. Jellinek). Classics of the alcohol literature: Scientific views of the spontaneous combustion of inebriates. *Quarterly Journal of Studies on Alcohol*, 1941, *2*, 804–805.

Engs, Ruth C. Let's look before we leap: The cognitive and behavioral evaluation of a university alcohol education program. *Journal of Alcohol and Drug Education*, 1977, *22*, 39–45.

Engs, Ruth C., and Fors, Stuart W. Drug abuse hysteria: The challenge of keeping perspective. *Journal of School Health*, 1988, *58*, 26–28.

Engs, Ruth C. Resurgence of a new "clean living" movement in the United States. *Journal of School Health*, 1991, *61*, 155–159.

Ennett, Susan T., Tobler, Nancy S., Ringwalt, Christopher L., and Flewelling, Robert L. How effective is Drug Abuse Resistance Education? A meta-analysis of Project DARE outcome evaluations. *American Journal of Public Health*, 1994, *84*, 1394–1401.

Erickson, Judith B. Making King Alcohol tremble. The juvenile work of the Women's Christian Temperance Union, 1874–1900. *Journal of Drug Education*, 1988, *18*, 333–352.

Ewing, John A., and Rouse, Beatrice A. Drinks, Drinkers, and Drinking. In: Ewing, John A., and Rouse, Beatrice A. (eds.) *Drinking: Alcohol in American Society—Issues and Current Research*. Chicago, IL: Nelson-Hall, 1978. pp. 5–30.

Famighetti, Robert (ed.) *The World Almanac and Book of Facts*. Mahwah, NJ: Funk & Wagnalls, 1995.

Feldman, Herman. *Prohibition: Its Economic and Industrial Aspects*. New York: D. Appleton and Co., 1928.

Ferrier, W. Kenneth. Alcohol Education in the Public School Curriculum. In: McCarthy, Raymond G. (ed.) *Alcohol Education for Classroom and Community*. New York: McGraw-Hill, 1964. pp. 48–68.

Fischer, Joseph M. A Comparison of Three Alcohol Education Instructional Approaches on the Attitudes and Knowledge of College Students. Unpublished Ph.D. dissertation, Oregon State University, 1990.

Flanders, Jessie K. *Legislative Control of the Elementary Curriculum*. New York: Teachers College, 1925.

Flanigan, Beverly. The hidden subverter: A case study in community adolescent alcohol education. *Journal of Alcohol and Drug Education*, 1987, *33*, 11–19.

Foerster, Louise. Influence of an Eighth-Grade Alcohol Education Program on Attitudes and Knowledge About Alcohol. Unpublished M.S. thesis, Arizona State University, 1985.

Ford, Gene. *The Benefits of Moderate Drinking: Alcohol, Health and Society*. San Francisco, CA: Wine Appreciation Guild, 1988.

Forney, Paul D., Forney, Mary A., and Ripley, William K. Alcohol and adolescents: Knowledge, attitudes, and behavior. *Journal of Adolescent Health Care*, 1988, *9*, 194–202.

Fullerton, M.S. Practical considerations for adopting, adapting and implementing alcohol/drug curriculums. *Journal of Alcohol and Drug Education*, 1983, *28*, 8–14.

Furnas, J. C. *The Life and Times of the Late Demon Rum*. New York: G. P. Putnam's Sons, 1965.

Gainer-Constine, Joanne. Evaluation of an Alcohol Education Curriculum Pilot Test. Unpublished M.S. thesis, University of Utah, 1984.

Garcia-McDonnell, Catherine L. The Effects of the Beginning Alcohol and Addictions Basic Education Studies (BABES) Prevention Curriculum on the Self-Esteem and Attitudes of Junior High School Students. Unpublished Ph.D. dissertation, Wayne State University, 1993.

General Accounting Office. *Drug Abuse Prevention: Federal Efforts To Identify Exemplary Programs Need Stronger Design.* Washington, DC: General Accounting Office, 1991.

George, Anthea. Why teaching kids to avoid peer pressure won't work. *Prevention Forum,* 1986, *6*, 2–4.

Georgia Department of Education. *Quality Core Curriculum, Health and Safety, K-12.* Atlanta, GA: Georgia Department of Education, n.d.

Gersick, Kerlin E., Grady, Katherine, and Snow, David L. Social-cognitive skill development with sixth graders and its initial impact on substance use. *Journal of Drug Education,* 1988, *18*, 55–70.

Gerstein, Dean R. Alcohol Use and Consequences. In: Moore, Mark H., and Gerstein, Dean R. (eds.) *Alcohol Use and Public Policy: Beyond the Shadow of Prohibition.* Washington, DC: National Academy Press, 1981. pp. 182–224.

Glassford, Darwin, Ivanoff, John, Sinsky, Anthony, and Pierce, Willard. Student generated solutions to the alcohol/drug problem. *Journal of Alcohol and Drug Education,* 1991, *37*, 65–71.

Glassner, Barry, and Berg, Bruce. Jewish-Americans and Alcohol: Processes of Avoidance and Definition. In: Bennett, Linda A., and Amers, Genevieve M. (eds.) *The American Experience with Alcohol: Contrasting Cultural Perspectives.* New York: Plenum, 1985. pp. 93–107.

Gliksman, Louis, Hart, David, Simpson, Robert, and Siess, Thomas. *Progress on Campus: Evaluation of the Campus Alcohol Policies and Education (CAPE) Program.* Toronto, Ontario, Canada: Addiction Research Foundation, 1987.

Gliksman, Louis, Douglas, Ronald R., and Smythe, Cindy. The impact of a high school alcohol education program utilizing a live theatrical performance: A comparitive study. *Journal of Drug Education,* 1983, *13*, 229–248.

Goldberg, P., and Meyers, E. J. The Influence of Public Understanding and Articles on Drug Education and Prevention. In: The Drug Abuse Council. *The Facts About Drug Abuse.* New York: Free Press, 1980. pp. 126–135.

Gonzalez, Gerardo M. The effect of a model alcohol education module on college students' attitudes, knowledge, and behavior related to alcohol use. *Journal of Alcohol and Drug Education,* 1980, *25*, 1–11.

Gonzalez, Gerardo M. Alcohol education can prevent alcohol problems: A summary of some unique research findings. *Journal of Alcohol and Drug Education,* 1982, *27*, 2–12.

Gonzales, Gerardo. Cited by Magner, D. K. Alcohol-related problems have not decreased on most college campuses survey indicates. *The Chronicle of Higher Education* (1988, November 9), A35, A37.

Gonzalez, Gerardo M. An integrated theoretical model for alcohol and other drug abuse prevention on the college campus. *Journal of College Student Development,* 1989, *30*, 492–503.

Gonzalez, Gerardo M. Effects of a theory-based, peer-focused drug education course. *Journal of Counseling and Development,* 1990, *68*, 446–449.

Goodstadt, Michael S. Shaping Drinking Practices Through Education. In: vonWartburg, Jean-Pierre, Magnenat, Pierre, Muller, Richard, and Wyss, Sonja (eds.) *Currents in Alcohol Research and the Prevention of Alcohol Problems: Proceedings of an International Symposium Held in Lausanne, Switzerland, November 7–9, 1983.* Berne, Switzerland: Hans Huber, 1985. pp. 85–106.

Goodstadt, Michael S. Alcohol education research and practice: A logical analysis of the two realities. *Journal of Drug Education*, 1986, *16*, 349–365.

Goodstadt, Michael S. Drug Education. *National Institute of Justice Crime File Study Guide*. Washington, DC: United States Department of Justice, 1988.

Goodstadt, Michael S., and Caleekal-John, Anuppa. Alcohol education programs for university students: A review of their effectiveness. *International Journal of the Addictions*, 1984, *19*, 721–741.

Goodstadt, Michael S., and Sheppard, Margaret. Three approaches to alcohol education. *Journal of Studies on Alcohol*, 1983, *44*, 362–380.

Goodstadt, Michael S., Sheppard, Margaret A., and Chan, Godwin C. An evaluation of two school-based alcohol education programs. *Journal of Studies on Alcohol*, 1982, *43*, 352–369.

Government Information Services. *Department of Education (Drug-Free Schools and Communities Act)*. Washington, DC: Government Information Services, 1991. (1991 Guide to Federal Funding for Anti-Drug Programs).

Grant, Marcus. Alcohol education: Does it really affect drinking problems? *Royal Society of Health Journal*, 1982, *102*, 201–204.

Grant, Marcus. Planning Effective Alcohol Education. In: Krasner, Neville, Madden, J. S., and Walker, Robin J. (eds.) *Alcohol Related Problems: Room for Manoeuvre*. New York: John Wiley & Sons, 1985. pp. 305–312.

Gray, Colleen B. Results of Alcohol Education for Junior High School Students: Utilitizing the Stanford D-E-C-I-D-E Alcohol Education Curriculum. Unpublished M.S. thesis, Southern Illinois University, 1984.

Greeley, Andrew M., McCready, William C., and Theisen, Gary. *Ethnic Drinking Subcultures*. New York: Praeger, 1980.

Green, Justin, and Kelley, John M. Evaluating the effectiveness of a school drug and alcohol prevention curriculum: A new look at "Here's Looking at You, Two." *Journal of Drug Education*, 1989, *19*, 117–132.

Gross, Leonard. *How Much Is Too Much?: The Effects of Social Drinking*. New York: Random House, 1983.

Gruber, Max. *Race Welfare*. Westerville, OH: American Issue Press, 1910.

Gusfield, Joseph R. *Symbolic Crusade: Status Politics and the American Temperance Movement*. Urbana, IL: University of Illinois Press, 1963.

Gusfield, Joseph R. Alcohol Problems—An Interactionist View. In: von Wartburg, Jean-Pierre, Magnenat, Pierre, Müller, Richard, and Wyss, Sonja (eds.) *Currents in Alcohol Research and the Prevention of Alcohol Problems—Proceedings of an International Symposium Held in Lausanne, Switzerland, November 7–9, 1983*. Berne, Switzerland: Hans Huber Publishers, 1985. pp. 71–81

Guthrie, R. S. Abstinence and Alcohol Use Among Senior Students Enrolled in Seventh-Day Adventist Academies. Unpublished M.S. thesis, University of Wisconsin-La Crosse, 1986.

Haines, Michael P. Eat, Drink and Be Merry: Signs and Symptoms of Alcohol Wellness. Paper presented at the American College Health Association annual meetings, St. Louis, MO, May 25–28, 1983. Educational Resources Information Center (ERIC) document number ED 238 850.

Hammond, Robert L. Elders sparks debate on legalization of drugs. *The Bottom Line on Alcohol In Society*, 1994, *15*, 5–15.

Hansen, William B., and Graham, John W. Preventing alcohol, marijuana, and cigarette use among adolescents: Peer pressure resistance training versus established conservative norms. *Preventive Medicine*, 1991, *20*, 414–430.

Hansen, William B., Johnson, C. Anderson, Flay, Brian R., Graham, John W., and Sobel, Judith. Affective and social influences approaches to the prevention of multiple substance abuse among seventh grade students: Results from Project SMART. *Preventive Medicine*, 1988, *17*, 135–154.

Hansen, William B., Malotte, C. Kevin, and Fielding, Jonathan E. Tobacco and alcohol prevention: Preliminary results of a four-year study. *Adolescent Psychiatry*, 1987, *14*, 556–575.

Hansen, William B., Malotte, C. Kevin, and Fielding, Jonathan E. Evaluation of a tobacco and alcohol abuse prevention curriculum for adolescents. *Health Education Quarterly*, 1988a, *15*, 93–114.

Hanson, David J. Dogmatism Among Specific Authoritarian and Non-Authoritarian Response Types. Unpublished M.A. thesis, Syracuse University, 1967.

Hanson, David J. Drug Education: Does It Work? In: Scarpitti, Frank R., and Datesman, Susan K. (eds.) *Drugs and the Youth Culture*. Beverly Hills, CA: Sage, 1980. pp. 251–282.

Hanson, David J. The Drinking Age Should be Lowered. In: Engs, Ruth C. (ed.) *Controversies in the Addictions Field*. Dubuque, IA: Kendall/Hunt, 1990. pp. 85–95. Reprinted in: Goldberg, Raymond (ed.) *Taking Sides: Clashing Views on Controversial Issues in Drugs and Society*. Guilford, CT: Dushkin, 1993. pp. 78–85.

Hanson, David J. *Preventing Alcohol Abuse: Alcohol, Culture, and Control*. Westport, CT: Praeger, 1995a.

Hanson, David J. The United States of America. In: Heath, Dwight B. (ed.) *International Handbook on Alcohol and Culture*. Westport, CT: Greenwood Press, 1995b. pp. 300–315.

Hanson, David J., and Engs, Ruth C. Drinking Behavior: Taking Personal Responsibility. In: Venturelli, Peter J. (ed.) *Drug Use in America: Social, Cultural, and Political Perspectives*. Boston, MA: Jones and Bartlett, 1994. pp. 175–181.

Hawaii State Department of Education. DARE Program Follow-Up Evaluation, 1988. Honolulu, HI: Hawaii State Department of Education, 1989. Educational Resources Information Center (ERIC) document number ED 311 325.

Heaney, Siobhan. An Evaluation of Alcohol Education in the School Setting. In: Krasner, Neville, Madden, J. S. and Walker, Robin J. (eds.) *Alcohol Related Problems: Room for Manoeuvre*. Chichester, England: John Wiley & Sons, 1984. pp. 313–319.

Heath, Dwight B. Drinking and drunkenness in transcultural perspective, Part II. *Transcultural Psychiatric Research Review*, 1986, *23*, 103–126.

Heath, Dwight B. A Decade of Development in the Anthropological Study of Alcohol Use: 1970–1980. In: Douglas, Mary (ed.) *Constructive Drinking: Perspectives on Drink from Anthropology*. New York: Cambridge University Press, 1987. pp. 16–69.

Heath, Dwight B. Quasi-science and public policy: A reply to Robin Room about details and misrepresentations in science. *Journal of Substance Abuse*, 1988b, *1*, 121–125.

Heath, Dwight, B. The new temperance movement: Through the looking glass. *Drugs and Society*, 1989, *3*, 143–168.

Heath, Dwight B. Flawed Policies from Flawed Premises: Pseudo-Science about Alcohol and Drugs. In: Engs, Ruth C. (ed.) *Controversies in the Addictions Field*, Vol. 1. Dubuque, IA: Kendall/Hunt, 1990. pp. 76–83.

Heien, Dale M., and Pittman, David J. The economic costs of alcohol abuse: An assessment of current methods and estimates. *Journal of Studies on Alcohol*, 1989, *50*, 567–579.

Heien, Dale M., and Pittman, David J. The external costs of alcohol abuse. *Journal of Studies on Alcohol*, 1993, *54*, 302–307.

Hennekens, C. H., Willett, W. Rosner, B., Cole, D. S., and Mayrent, S. L. Effects of beer, wine, and liquor on coronary deaths. *Journal of the American Medical Association*, 1979, *242*, 1973–1974.

Hofstader, Richard. *The Age of Reform: From Bryan to F.D.R.*. New York: Vintage, 1965.

Homel, Peter J., Daniels, Philip, Reid, Thomas R., and Lawson, James S. Results of an experimental school-based health development programme in Australia. *International Journal of Health Education*, 1981, *24*, 263–270.

Hopkins, Ronald H., Mauss, Armand, Kearney, Kathleen A., and Weisheit, Ralph A. Comprehensive evaluation of a model alcohol education curriculum. *Journal of Studies on Alcohol*, 1988, *49*, 38–50.

Horan, John J., and Williams, John M. Longitudinal study of assertion training as a drug abuse strategy. *American Educational Research Journal*, 1982, *19*, 341–351.

Horton, Lowell. The education of most worth: Preventing drug and alcohol abuse. *Educational Leadership*, 1988, *45*, 4–8.

Horton, Lowell. Don't let drug programs send deadly messages. *The Education Digest*, 1989, *54*, 38–39.

Horton, Lowell. *Developing Effective Drug Education Programs*. Bloomington, IN: Phi Delta Kappa Educational Foundation, 1992.

Howe, Barbara. *Alcohol Education: A Handbook for Health and Welfare Professionals*. London, England: Tavistock/Routledge, 1989.

Hunt, Mary H. *A History of the First Decade of the Department of Scientific Temperance Instruction in Schools and Colleges* Boston, MA: Washington Press, 1892.

Hunt, Mary H. *An Epoch of the Nineteenth Century: An Outline of the Work for Scientific Temperance Education in the Public Schools of the United States*. Boston, MA: Foster, 1897.

Hunt, Mary H. *Reply to the Physiological Subcommittee of the Committee of Fifty*. Washington, DC: 58th Congress, 2nd Session. Senate Document No. 171, 1904.

Hyman, Merton, Zimmerman, Marilyn, Gurioli, Carol, and Helrich, Alice. *Drinkers, Drinking and Alcohol-Related Mortality and Hospitalization*. New Brunswick, NJ: Rutgers Center for Alcohol Studies, 1980.

Inciardi, J. A. *The War on Drugs: Heroin, Cocaine, Crime, and Public Policy*. Palo Alto, CA: Mayfield, 1986.

Institute for Social Research. Monitoring the Future Questionnare. Ann Arbor, MI: The University of Michigan, Institute for Social Research, 1986.

Irwin, Darrell D. The Effects of Campus Alcohol and Drug Prevention Programs on the Behaviors of University Students. Unpublished Ph.D. dissertation, Loyola University of Chicago, 1994.

Isaac, Paul E. *Prohibition and Politics: Turbulent Decades in Tennessee, 1885–1920*. Knoxville, TN: University of Tennessee Press, 1965.

Jackson, Valera M., Dorman, Steve M., Tennant, L. Keith, and Chen, William W. The Effects of teaching specific guidelines for alcohol consumption on alcohol knowledge and behavioral intent of college students. *Health Education*, 1989, *20*, 51–54.

Jaschik, S. Investigators to visit campuses to check for illegal drug use. *The Chronicle of Higher Education*, 1989 (April), A1, A26.

Jensen, Margaret, Wakat, Diane, Gansneder, Bruce, and Paviour, Peggy B. Student desires for a university drug education program. *Journal of Drug Education*, 1989, *19*, 231–244.

Jessor, Richard, Young, H. B., Young, E. B., and Teri, C. Perceived opportunity, alienation, and drinking behavior among Italian and American youth. *Journal of Personality and Social Psychology*, 1970, *15*, 215–222.

Johnson, C. Anderson, Pentz, Mary A., Weber, Mark D., Dwyer, James H., Baer, Neal, MacKinnon, David P., Hansen, William B., and Flay, Brian R. Relative effectiveness of comprehensive community programming for drug abuse prevention with high-risk and low-risk adolescents. *Journal of Consulting and Clinical Psychology*, 1990, *58*, 447–456.

Johnson, Elaine M., Amatetti, Sharon, Funkhouser, Judith E., and Johnson, Sandie. Theories and models supporting prevention approaches to alcohol problems among youth. *Public Health Reports*, 1988, *103*, 578–586.

Johnson, Timmy D. An Assessment of the Effectiveness of a Suburban Police Department's Project DARE (Drug Abuse Resistance Education) Program on Student Knowledge of Drugs, Alcohol, and Tobacco. Unpublished Ed.D. dissertation, Wayne State University, 1994.

Jorgensen, Leeann. College Alcohol and Drug Prevention Program: An Evaluation. Unpublished Ph.D. dissertation, Union Institute, 1990.

Kallmeyer, K. Erfahrungen uber aufklarungsaktionen zum rauschmittel-, raucher-, und alkohol problem in schulen. *Offentliche Gesundheitswesen*, 1980, *42*, 251–254.

Katcher, Brian S. Benjamin Rush's educational campaign against hard drinking. *American Journal of Public Health*, 1993, *83*, 273–281.

Keller, J. Why People Drink. Presentation to College of Education faculty, Michigan State University, 1979.

Keller, Mark. Alcohol Problems and Policies. In: Kyvig, David E. (ed.) *Law, Alcohol, and Order*. Westport, CT: Greenwood Press, 1985. pp.159–175.

Kennedy, Patrick J. The Effect of Moderate Drinking Skill Training on Alcohol Related Knowledge, Attitude, and Behavior. Unpublished Ph.D. dissertation, University of Minnesota, 1989.

Kenney, P. W. Prospective teachers' attitudes toward alcohol education. *Journal of Alcohol and Drug Education*, 1978, *24*, 14–30.

Kerr, K. Austin. *Organized for Prohibition: A New History of the Anti-Saloon League.* New Haven, CT: Yale University Press, 1985.

Kim, Sehwan. A short- and long-term evaluation of Here's Looking at You alcohol education program. *Journal of Drug Education*, 1988, *18*, 235–242.

Klee, Thomas E. The Effectiveness of a Model Drug and Alcohol Abuse Prevention Program on Low-Risk Students. Unpublished Ph.D. dissertation, Temple University, 1982.

Kobler, John. *Ardent Spirits: The Rise and Fall of Prohibition.* New York: G.P. Putnam's Sons, 1973.

Kozarerevic, D. J., Vojvodie, N., Dawber, T., McGee, G., Racic, Z., Gordon, T., and Zukel, W. Frequency of alcohol consumption and morbidity and mortality. *Lancet*, 1980, *1:8169*, 613–616.

Kreutter, Karole J., Gewirtz, Herbert, Davenny, Joan E., and Love, Carol. Drug and alcohol prevention project for sixth graders: First-year findings. *Adolescence*, 1991, *26*, 287–293.

Krout, John A. *The Origins of Prohibition.* New York: Knopf, 1925.

Kuehn, Ann M. An Application of the Social Cognitive Theory in Comparing the Effectiveness of a Peer-Led Versus a Staff-Led On-Campus Alcohol Education Program. Unpublished M.Ed. thesis, University of Nebraska, 1991.

Kyvig, David E. *Repealing National Prohibition.* Chicago, IL: University of Chicago Press, 1979.

Kyvig, David E. Sober Thoughts: Myths and Realities on National Prohibition after Fifty Years. In: Kyvig, David E. (ed.) *Law, Alcohol, and Order: Perspectives on National Prohibition.* Westport, CT: Greenwood Press, 1985. pp. 3–20.

La Piere, Richard T. Attitudes vs. actions. *Social Forces*, 1934, *13*, 230–237.

Lasswell, H. D., and Rubenstein, R. *The Sharing of Power in a Psychiatric Hospital*. New Haven, CT: Yale University Press, 1966.

Lavik, Nils J. The Akershus project: Development and evaluation of three programs of drug and alcohol education in junior high schools. *Journal of Alcohol and Drug Education*, 1986, *32*, 47–62.

Lee, Alfred M. Techniques of social reform: An analysis of the New Prohibition Drive. *American Sociological Review*, 1944, *9*, 65–77. Reprinted as the New Prohibition Drive. In: McCarthy, Raymond G. (ed.) *Drinking and Intoxication: Selected Readings in Social Attitudes and Controls*. New Haven, CT: College and University Press, 1959. pp. 412–428.

Lender, Mark E., and Martin, James K. *Drinking in America: A History*. New York: The Free Press, 1982.

Levine, Harry G. The alcohol problem in America: From temperance to alcoholism. *British Journal of Addiction*, 1984, *79*, 109–119.

Levine, Harry. The birth of American alcohol control: Prohibition, the lawlessness. *Contemporary Drug Problems*, 1985, *12*, 63–115.

Lignell, Constance, and Davidhizer, Ruth. Effect of drug and alcohol education on attitudes of high school students. *Journal of Drug and Alcohol Education*, 199, *37*, 31–37.

Liska, A. E. (ed.) *The Consistency Controversy*. New York: John Wiley, 1975.

Lobello, Steven G., Tarpley, Bayard S., and Day, Charles L. Credibility of sources of information about alcohol among high school students. *Journal of Alcohol and Drug Education*, 1988, *33*, 68–72.

Logan, Nancy J. The Effects of an Alcohol Education Program on the Alcohol Knowledge of Underclassmen at Southern Illinois University at Carbondale. Unpublished M.S. thesis, Southern Illinois University, 1980.

Lolli, Georgio, Serianni, Emidic, Golden, Grace M., and Luzzatto-Fegiz, Pierpeolo. *Alcohol in Italian Culture: Food and Wine in Relation to Sobriety Among Italians and Italian Americans*. Glencoe, IL: Free Press, 1958.

London, William M., and Duquette, R. Daniel. Does "activated" alcohol education reduce disruptive drinking behavior among university students? *Health Education*, 1989, *20*, 30–34.

LoSciuto, Leonard, and Ausetts, Mary A. Evaluation of a drug abuse prevention program: A field experiment. *Addictive Behaviors*, 1988, *13*, 337–351.

Lotterhos, J. F., Glover, E. D., Holbert, D., and Barnes, R. C. Intentionality of college students regarding North Carolina's 21-year drinking age law. *International Journal of Addiction*, 1988, *23*, 629–647.

MacAndrew, Craig, and Edgerton, Robert B. *Drunken Comportment: A Social Explanation*. Chicago, IL: Aldine, 1969.

MacKinnon, David P., Johnson, C. Anderson, Pentz, Mary A., Dwyer, James H., Hansen, William B., Flay, Brian R., and Wang, Eric Yu-I. Mediating mechanisms in a school-based drug prevention program: First-year effects of the Midwestern Prevention Project. *Health Psychology*, 1991, *10*, 164–172.

Mahaffey, James M. A Study to Determine the Increase in Knowledge of Drugs and Drug Abuse by Fourth-Graders as a Result of the "Here's Looking at You Two" Drug and Alcohol Abuse Education Curriculum. Unpublished Ph.D. dissertation, University of South Carolina, 1988.

Maine State Department of Education. Leadership in Maine. (Poster) Augusta, ME: Maine State Department of Education, n.d.

Malvin, Janet H., Moskowitz, Joel M., Schaps, Eric, and Schaeffer, Gary A. Evaluation of two school-based alternatives programs. *Journal of Alcohol and Drug Education*, 1985, *30*, 98–109.

Manley Drug Education and Counselling Centre. *The Responsible Use of Alcohol: Results of a Pilot Study*. Manley, New South Wales, Australia: Manley Drug Education and Counselling Centre, 1987.

Marshall, Mac (ed.) *Beliefs, Behaviors, & Alcoholic Beverages: A Cross-Cultural Survey*. Ann Arbor, MI: University of Michigan Press, 1979.

Marshall, Mac. Conclusions. In: Marshall, Mac (ed.) *Beliefs, Behaviors, and Alcoholic Beverages: A Cross-Cultural Survey*. Ann Arbor, MI: University of Michigan Press, 1979. pp. 451–457.

May, Carl. Resistance to peer group pressure: An inadequate basis for alcohol education. *Health Education Research*, 1993, *8*, 159–165.

McAlister, Alfred, Perry, Cheryl, Killen, Joel, Slinkard, Lee A., and Maccoby, Nathan. Pilot study of smoking, alcohol, and drug abuse prevention. *American Journal of Public Health*, 1980, *70*, 719–721.

McCarthy, Raymond G. Editorial introduction to chapter three. In: McCarthy, Raymond G. (ed.) *Drinking and Intoxication: Selected Readings in Social Attitudes and Controls*. New Haven, CT: College and University Press, 1959. p. 26.

McCarthy, Raymond G., and Douglass, Edgar M. *Alcohol and Social Responsibility: A New Educational Approach*. New York: Thomas Y. Crowell and Yale Plan Clinic, 1949.

McConnell, D. W. Temperance Movements. In: Seligman, Edwin R. A., and Johnson, Alvin (eds.) *Encyclopedia of the Social Sciences*. New York, NY: The Macmillan Co., 1963.

McGranor, Diane. The Effect of Education on Adolescents Regarding Their Knowledge in the Use of Alcohol, Smoking, and Nutrition on the Outcome of Pregnancy. Unpublished M.S. thesis, State University of New York at Buffalo, 1982.

McKnight, A. James, and McPherson, Kenard. Evaluation of peer intervention training for high school alcohol safety education. *Accident Analysis and Prevention*, 1986, *18*, 339–347.

McManus, Mary M. Pilot Study of the Short Term Effects of Three Methods of Alcohol Education on Selected Student Groups at Western Wisconsin Technical Institute. Unpublished M.S. thesis, University of Wisconsin at La Crosse, 1980.

McNamara-Meis, Kathy. Burned. *Forbes MediaCritic*, 1995, 20–24.

McPherson, Kenard, McKnight, A. James, Weidman, J. R. *Supplemental Driver Safety Program Development: Final Report, Vol. 1, Developmental Research and Evaluation*. Prepared for DOT/NHTSA under Contract No. DOT-HS-9-02284, February 1983.

Meacci, William G. An evaluation of the effects of college alcohol education on the prevention of negative consequences. *Journal of Alcohol and Drug Education*, 1990, *35*, 66–72.

Meeks, L., and Heit, P. *Health 6: Focus on You*. Columbus, OH: Merrell, 1986.

Mendelson, Jack H., and Mello, Nancy K. *Alcohol: Use and Abuse in America*. Boston, MA: Little, Brown & Co., 1985.

Merz, Charles. *The Dry Decade*. Seattle, WA: University of Washington Press, 1969. (Contains a new introduction by the author. Originally published in 1930.)

A Methodist editor. *The American Issue*, 1970 (January) quoted by Kobler, John. *Ardent Spirits*. New York: G.P. Putnam's Sons, 1973.

Mezvinsky, Norton. The White Ribbon Reform, 1874–1920. Unpublished Ph.D. dissertation, University of Wisconsin, 1959.

Mezvinsky, Norton. Scientific temperance instruction in the schools. *History of Education Quarterly*, 1961, *1*, 48–56.

Mielke, Dan, and Holstedt, Peggy. *Oregon Alcohol and Drug Prevention Education (ADADE) Infused Lesson Guide, K12*. Salem, OR: Oregon Department of Education and Eastern Oregon State College, 1991.

Milgram, Gail G. A historical review of alcohol education research and comments. *Journal of Alcohol and Drug Education*, 1976, *22*, 1–16.

Miller, II, Donald N. The Effects of Two Methodological Approaches in Alcohol Education on the Knowledge, Attitudes, and Behaviors of College Students. Unpublished Ph.D. dissertation, Pennsylvania State University, 1982.

Miller, Ramona L. Positive self-esteem and alcohol/drug related attitudes among school children. *Journal of Alcohol and Drug Education*, 1988, *33*, 26–31.

Miron, Jeffrey, and Zweibel, Jeffrey. Alcohol consumption during prohibition. *American Economic Review: Papers and Proceedings*, 1991, *81*, 242–247.

Mitchell, Margaret E., Hu, Teh-Wei, McDonnell, Nancy S., and Swisher, John D. Cost-effectiveness analysis of an educational drug abuse prevention program. *Journal of Drug Education*, 1984, *14*, 271–292.

Modell, Walter. Mass drug catastrophes and the roles of science and technology. *Science*, 1967, *156*, 346–351.

Moore, Mark H. Actually, prohibition was a success. *New York Times*, 1989 (October 16), p. A-21.

Moore, Merrill. The alcohol problem in the military service. *Quarterly Journal of Studies on Alcohol*, 1942, *3*, 244–256.

Morgan, Patricia. Industrialization, urbanization, and the attack on Italian drinking culture. *Contemporary Drug Problems*, 1988, *15*, 607–626.

Morton, Mary B. *Criteria for the Development or Selection of Drug Prevention Curricula*. Atlanta, GA: Southeast Regional Center for Drug-Free Schools and Communities, 1990.

Mosher, James F. The History of Youthful-Drinking Laws: Implications for Current Policy. In: Wechsler, Henry (ed.) *Minimum-Drinking-Age Laws: An Evaluation*. Lexington, MA: Lexington Books, 1980. pp. 11–38.

Moskowitz, Joel M. The primary prevention of alcohol problems: A critical review of the research literature. *Journal of Studies on Alcohol*, 1989, *50*, 54–88.

Moskowitz, Joel M., Malvin, Janet H., Schaeffer, Gary A., and Schaps, Eric. Evaluation of a junior high school primary prevention program. *Addictive Behaviors*, 1983, *8*, 393–401.

Moskowitz, Joel M., Schaps, Eric, Malvin, Janet H., and Schaeffer, Gary A. The effects of a drug education at follow-up. *Journal of Alcohol and Drug Education*, 1984a, *30*, 45–49.

Moskowitz, Joel M., Malvin, Janet H., Schaeffer, Gary A., and Schaps, Eric. An experimental evaluation of a drug education course. *Journal of Drug Education*, 1984b, *14*, 9–21.

Mulford, Harold A. The Epidemiology of Alcoholism and Its Implications. In: Pattison, E. Mansell, and Kaufman, Edward (eds.) *Encyclopedic Handbook of Alcoholism*. New York: Gardner Press, 1982. pp. 441–457.

Mulford, Harold A. What I would most like to know. What if alcoholism had not been invented? The dynamics of American alcohol mythology. *Addiction*, 1994, *89*, 517–520.

Mulford, Harold A., Ledolter, J., and Fitzgerald, J. L. Alcohol availability and consumption: Iowa sales data revisited. *Journal of Studies on Alcohol*, 1992, *53*, 487–494.

Mulford, Harold A., Ledolter, J., and Fitzgerald, J. L. Scientific discovery or reality construction? A response to Wagenaar and Holder. *Journal of Studies on Alcohol*, 1993, *54*, 252–253.

Mullin, I. S. Alcohol education: The school's responsibility. *Journal of School Health*, 1968, *38*, 518–522.

Nathan, Peter E. Failures in prevention: Why we can't prevent the devastating effect of alcoholism and drug abuse? *American Psychologist*, 1983, *38*, 459–467.

National Commission on Marijuana and Drug Abuse. *Drug Use in America: Problem in Perspective*. Washington, DC: Government Printing Office, 1973.

National Institute on Alcohol Abuse and Alcoholism. *Alcohol and Health: Third Special Report to the U.S. Congress*. Rockville, MD: National Institute on Alcohol Abuse and Alcoholism, 1978.

National Temperance and Prohibition Council. *1991 Resolutions*. Evanston, IL: National Temperance and Prohibition Council, 1991.

National Temperance and Prohibition Council. *National Leadership Specializing on Alcohol Issues*. (Pamphlet) Evanston, IL: National Temperance and Prohibition Council, n.d.

Newman, Ian M., Anderson, Carolyn S., and Farrell, Katherine A. Role reversal and efficacy: Two 15-month evaluations of a ninth-grade alcohol education program. *Journal of Drug Education*, 1992, *22*, 55–67.

Newman, Ian M., Mohr, Patricia, Badger, Barbara, and Gillespie, Timothy S. Effects of teacher preparation and student age on an alcohol and drug education curriculum. *Journal of Drug Education*, 1984, *14*, 23–36.

New York State Division of Alcoholism and Alcohol Abuse. *Alcohol; The Gateway Drug*. Albany, NY: New York State Division of Alcoholism and Alcohol Abuse, n.d.a.

New York State Division of Alcoholism and Alcohol Abuse. Do You Use Drugs? (Poster) Albany, NY: New York State Division of Alcoholism and Alcohol Abuse, n.d.b.

New York State Division of Alcoholism and Alcohol Abuse. Don't be Fooled. (Poster) Albany, NY: New York State Division of Alcoholism and Alcohol Abuse, n.d.c.

Nietz, John A. *Old Textbooks: Spelling, Grammar, Reading, Arithmetic, Geography, American History, Civil Government, Physiology, Penmanship, Art, Music—Taught in the Common Schools From Colonial Days to 1900*. Pittsburgh, PA: University of Pittsburgh Press, 1961.

O'Connor, John, and Saunders, Bill. Drug education: An appraisal of a popular preventive. *International Journal of the Addictions*, 1992, *27*, 165–185.

Odegard, Peter H. *Pressure Politics: The Story of the Anti-Saloon League*. New York: Columbia University Press, 1928.

Office for Substance Abuse Prevention. *Be Smart! Don't Start! Just Say No!* Rockville, MD: Office for Substance Abuse Prevention, 1987.

Office for Substance Abuse Prevention. *What You Can Do About Drug Use in America*. Rockville, MD: Office for Substance Abuse Prevention, 1988.

Office for Substance Abuse Prevention. *Alcohol, Tobacco, and Other Drugs Resource Guide*. Rockville, MD: Office for Substance Abuse Prevention, 1993.

Ohles, John F. The imprimatur of Mary H. H. Hunt. *Journal of School Health*, 1978, *48*, 477–478.

Ormond, Charl. *Temperance Education in American Public Schools*. Westerville, OH: American Issue Press, 1929.

Page, C. The new sobriety's thirst for virtue. *Washington Times*, (January 9). 1991.

Palmer, Carolyn J., Gehring, Donald D., and Guthrie, Victoria L. Student knowledge of information mandated by the 1989 amendments to the Drug Free Schools and Communities Act. *NASPA Journal*, 1992, *30*, (30–38).

Palmer, S. E. House votes to bar education department funds from colleges that lack drug-abuse programs. *The Chronicle of Higher Education* 1986 (October 6), A1.

Parker, Douglas A. Alcohol Control Policy in the United States. In: Miller, Peter M., and Nirenberg, Ted D. (eds.) *Prevention of Alcohol Abuse*. New York: Plenum Press, 1984. pp. 235–244.

Pauly, Philip, J. The struggle for ignorance about alcohol: American physiologists, Wilbur Olin Atwater, and the Women's Christian Temperance Union. *Bulletin of the History of Medicine*, 1990, *64*, 366–392.

Peele, Stanton. The limitations of control-of-supply models for explaining and preventing alcoholism and drug addiction. *Journal of Studies on Alcohol*, 1987, *48*, 61–77.

Peele, Stanton. *Diseasing of America: Addiction Treatment out of Control*. Lexington, MA: Lexington Books, 1989.

Pentz, Mary A., Dwyer, James H., MacKinnon, David P., Flay, Brian R., Hansen, William B., Wang, E., and Johnson, C. Anderson. A multi-community trial for primary prevention of adolescent drug abuse: Effects on drug use prevalence. *Journal of the American Medical Association*, 1989, *261*, 3259–3266.

Perry, Cheryl L. Prevention of alcohol use and abuse in adolescence: Teacher- vs peer-led intervention. *Crisis*, 1989, *10*, 52–61.

Pipher, James R., and Rivers, Clayton. The differential effects of alcohol education on junior high school students. *Journal of Alcohol and Drug Education*, 1982, *27*, 73–88.

Pittman, David J. *Primary Prevention of Alcohol Abuse and Alcoholism: An Evaluation of the Control of Consumption Policy*. St. Louis, MO: Washington University, Social Science Institute, 1980.

Plaut, Thomas F. A. *Alcohol Problems: A Report to the Nation by the Cooperative Commission on the Study of Alcoholism*. New York, NY: Oxford University Press, 1967.

Plaut, Thomas F. A. Prevention of Alcoholism. In: Golann, S.F., and Eisdorfer, C. (eds.) *Handbook of Community Mental Health*. New York: Appleton-Century-Crofts, 1972. pp. 421–438.

Ploetz, Alfred J. *The Influence of Alcohol Upon the Race*. Westerville, OH: American Issue Press, 1915.

Polich, J. M., Ellickson, P., Reuter, P., and Kahan, J. *Strategies for Controlling Adolescent Drug Use*. Santa Monica, CA: Rand Corp., 1984.

Pollard, Joseph P. *The Road to Repeal: Submission to Conventions*. New York: Brentano's , 1932, p. 107. Cited by Sinclair, Andrew. *Prohibition: The Era of Excess*. Boston: Little, Brown & Co., 1962, p. 110.

Popham, Robert E. The Social History of the Tavern. In: Israel, Yedy, Glaser, Frederick B., Kalant, Harold, Popham, Robert E., Schmidt, Harold, and Smart, Reginald G. (eds.) *Research Advances in Alcohol and Drug Problems*. New York: Plenum, 1978. Volume 4. pp. 255–302.

Portnoy, Barry. Effects of a controlled-usage alcohol education program based on the health belief model. *Journal of Drug Education*, 1980, *10*, 181–195.

Prendergast, Michael L. A History of Alcohol Problem Prevention Efforts in the United States. In: Holder, Harold D. (ed.) *Control Issues on Alcohol Abuse Prevention: Strategies for States and Communities*. Greenwich, CT: JAI Press, 1987. pp. 25–52.

Presley, Cheryl, Harrold, Roger, Scouten, Eric, and Lyeria, Rob. *Core Pre/Post Evaluation Instrument User's Manual*. Carbondale, IL: The Core Institute, 1990.

Rapaport, Ross J., Minelli, Mark J., Reyes, Sally, and Norton, Penny. Involving recovering students and community members in alcohol and other drug-abuse prevention. *Journal of College Student Development*, 1994, *35*, 136–137.

Reall, Jennifer L. A Comparison of Drinking Attitudes and Behavior Between Selected Participating and Non-Participating Residence Hall Students in a Voluntary Alcohol Education Program at Mankato State University. Unpublished M.S. thesis, Mankato State University, 1989.

Ringwalt, Christopher, Ennett, Susan T., and Holt, Kathleen D. An outcome evaluation of Project DARE (Drug Abuse Resistance Education). *Health Education Research*, 1991, *6*, 327–337.

Ripley, George, and Dana, Charles A. (eds.). *The New American Cyclopaedia: A Popular Dictionary of General Knowledge*. New York: D. Appleton and Co., 1857. Volume 1.

Robbins, Michael C. Problem-Drinking and the Integration of Alcohol in Rural Buganda. In: Marshall, Mac (ed.) *Beliefs, Behaviors, & Alcoholic Beverages: A Cross-Cultural Survey*. Ann Arbor, MI: University of Michigan Press, 1979. pp. 362–379.

Robinson, III, James. The Effects of Three Alcohol Education Instruction Programs on the Knowledge, Attitudes, and Drinking Behaviors of College Students. Unpublished Ed.D. dissertation, University of Northern Colorado, 1980.

Robinson, III, James. A comparison of three alcohol instruction programs on the knowledge, attitudes, and drinking behaviors of college students. *Journal of Drug Education*, 1981, *11*, 157–166.

Robinson, R. R. The prospect of adequate education about alcohol and alcoholism. *Journal of Alcohol Education*, 1969, *14*, 1–4.

Robinson, Sharon E., Roth Sari, L., Gloria, Alberta M., Keim, Jean, and Sattler, Howard. Influence of substance abuse education on undergraduates' knowledge, attitudes, and behaviors. *Journal of Drug And Alcohol Education*, 1993, *39*, 123–130.

Roizen, Ron. Redefining alcohol in post-repeal America: Lessons from the short life of Everett Colby's Council for Moderation, 1934–1936. *Contemporary Drug Problems*, 1991, *18*, 237–272.

Room, Robin. The Prevention of Alcohol Problems. Berkeley, CA: Social Research Group, 1977. Social Research Group Working Paper F–63. Quoted in Wallack, Lawrence M. Mass media campaigns: The odds against finding behavior changes. *Health Education Quarterly*, 1981, *8*, 209–260.

Room, Robin. Alcohol as a Course: Empirical Links and Social Definitions. In: von Wartburg, Jean-Pierre, Magnenat, Pierre, Müller, Richard, and Wyss, Sonja (eds.) *Currents in Alcohol Research and the Prevention of Alcohol Problems: Proceedings of an International Symposium Held in Lausanne, Switzerland, November 7–9, 1983*. Berne, Switzerland: Hans Huber, 1985. pp. 11–19.

Room, Robin. Science is in the details: Towards a nuanced view of alcohol control studies. *Journal of Substance Abuse*, 1988, *1*, 117–120.

Room, Robin. Cultural Changes in Drinking and Trends in Alcohol Problem Indicators: Recent U.S. Experience. In: Clark, Walter B., and Hilton, Michael E. (eds.) *Alcohol in America: Drinking Practices and Problems*. Albany, NY: State University of New York Press, 1991. pp. 149–162.

Rorabaugh, William J. *The Alcoholic Republic: An American Tradition*. New York: Oxford University Press, 1979.

Rorabaugh, William J. Alcohol in America. *OAH Magazine of History*, 1991, *6*, 17–19.

Rorabaugh, William J. Alcohol and Alcoholism. In: Cayton, Mark K., Gorn, Elliott J., and Williams, Peter W. (eds.) *Encyclopedia of American Social History*. New York: Charles Scribner's Sons, 1993. Volume 3. pp. 2135–2142.

Ross, H. Laurence, and Hughes, Graham. Getting MADD in vain: Drunk driving—what not to do. *The Nation*, 1986, *243*, 663–664.

Ross, H. Lawrence. Reflections on doing policy-relevant sociology: How to cope with MADD mothers. *The American Sociologist*, 1987, *18*, 173–177.

Rostow, Eugene V. Recent proposals for federal legislation controlling the use of liquor. *Quarterly Journal of Studies on Alcohol*, 1942, *3*, 230–235.

Roueché, Berton. *The Neutral Spirit: A Portrait of Alcohol*. Boston: Little, Brown & Co., 1960.

Roueché, Berton. Alcohol in Human Culture. In: Lucia, Salvatore P. (ed.) *Alcohol and Civilization*. New York: McGraw-Hill, 1963. pp. 167–182.

Royce, James E. *Alcohol Problems and Alcoholism: A Comprehensive Survey*. New York: Free Press, 1981.

Rozelle, George R. Experential and cognitive small group approaches to alcohol education for college students. *Journal of Alcohol and Drug Education*, 1980, *26*, 40–54.

Rubin, Jay L. The Wet War: American Liquor Control, 1941–1945. In: Blocker, Jr., Jack S. (ed.) *Alcohol, Reform and Society: The Liquor Issue in Social Context*. Westport, CT: Greenwood Press, 1979. pp. 235–258. Contributions in American History, Number 83.

St. Pierre, Richard, and Miller, Donald N. Future directions for school-based alcohol education. *Health Education*, 1986, *6*, 11–13.

Salvagnini, M., Gallimberti, L., Benussi, G., Del Borello, A., Dell'Oro, A., Orlandini, D., Piccoli, A., Ricci, G. P., Sciarrone, R., and Naccarato, R. Evaluation of a structured alcohol education course in a secondary school system in North Italy. *Drug And Alcohol Dependence*, 1983, *12,* 181–188.

Sarvela, Paul D., and McClendon, E. J. An impact evaluation of a rural youth drug education program. *Journal of Drug Education*, 1987, *17*, 213–231.

Schach, Margaret A. An Analysis of a Sixth Grade Alcohol and Drug Education Program. Unpublished M.S. thesis, Western Illinois University, 1990.

Schaps, Eric, Moskowitz, Joel M., Condon, John W., and Malvin, Janet H. Process and outcome evaluation of a drug education course. *Journal of Drug Education*, 1982, *12*, 353–364.

Schlaadt, Richard G. *Alcohol Use and Abuse*. Guilford, CT: Dushkin Publishing, 1992.

Schlegel, Ronald P., Manske, Stephen R., and Page, Andrea. A Guided Decision-Making Programs for Elementary School Students: A Field Experiment in Alcohol Education. In: Miller, Peter M., and Nirenberg, Ted D. (eds.) *Prevention of Alcohol Abuse*. New York, NY: Plenum Press, 1984. pp. 407–439.

Schmidt, Laura A. "A battle not man's but God's": Origins of the American temperance crusade in the struggle for religious authority. *Journal of Studies on Alcohol*, 1995, *56*, 110–121.

Schmidt, Wolfgang. Regulating the Supply of Alcoholic Beverages—A New Concept for an Old Ideology? In: von Wartburg, Jean-Pierre, Magnenat, Pierre, Müller, Richard, and Wyss, Sonja (eds.) *Currents in Alcohol Research and the Prevention of Alcohol Problems: Proceedings of an International Symposium Held in Lausanne, Switzerland, November 7–9, 1983*. Berne, Switzerland: Hans Huber, 1985. pp. 107–118.

Schwartz, R. Rethinking the "failures" of prohibition. *U.S. Journal of Alcohol & Drug Dependence*, 1990, *14*, 5.

Seif, Mary J. A Self-Esteem Approach to Social Success and Alcohol/Drug Prevention for Fourth Grade Students. Unpublished M.Ed. thesis, Ashland University, 1990.

Seldes, George (compiler). *The Great Quotations*. New York: Lyle Stuart, 1960.

Sewall, Thomas. *Effects of Intemperance on the Intellectual, Moral and Physical Powers.* Albany, NY: 1841. Quoted by Krout, John A. *The Origins of Prohibition.* New York: Alfred A. Knopf, 1925, p. 229.

Sheehan, Nancy M. The WCTU and education: Canadian-American illustrations. *Journal of the Midwest History of Education Society*, 1981, *9*, 115–133.

Sheehan, Nancy M. The WCTU and educational strategies on the Canadian prairie. *History of Education Quarterly*, 1984a, *24*, 101–119.

Sheehan, Nancy M. National pressure groups and provincial curriculum policy: Temperance in Nova Scotia schools 1880–1930. *Canadian Journal of Education*, 1984b, *9*, 73–88.

Shepherd, William G. *Colliers Weekly*, July 26, 1930. Cited by Asbury, Herbert. *The Great Illusion: An Informed History of Prohibition.* New York: Doubleday & Co., 1950.

Shope, Jean T., Dielman, T. E., Butchart, Amy T., Campanelli, Pamela C., and Kloska, Deborah D. An elementary school-based alcohol misuse prevention program: A follow-up evaluation. *Journal of Studies on Alcohol*, 1992, *53*, 106–121.

Shope, Jean T., Kloska, Deborah D., Dielman, T. E., and Maharg, Ruth. Longitudinal evaluation of an enhanced alcohol misuse prevention study (AMPS) curriculum for grades six–eight. *Journal of School Health*, 1994, *64*, 160–166.

Simpson, Jeff. A Comparison of Two Approaches to Alcohol Education. Unpublished M.S. thesis, Western Illinois University, 1979.

Sinclair, Andrew. *Prohibition: The Era of Excess.* Boston, MA: Little, Brown & Co., 1962.

Single, Eric W. The Availability Theory of Alcohol-Related Problems. In: Chaudron, C. Douglas, and Wilkinson, D. Adrian (eds.) *Theories on Alcoholism.* Toronto, Ontario: Addiction Research Foundation, 1988. pp. 325–351.

Smith, Marcus. *The Boston Speaker.* Boston, MA: Joseph Dowe, 6th ed., 1844. Cited by Elson, Ruth M. in *Guardians of Tradition: American Schoolbooks of the Nineteenth Century.* Lincoln, NE: University of Nebraska Press, 1964, p. 319.

Snowden, Lynn. . . . and make mine a double: When did social drinking become such a faux pas? *Utne Reader*, 1992, *51*, 130–131.

Snyder, Charles R. *Alcohol and the Jews: A Cultural Study of Drinking and Sobriety.* Glencoe, IL: Free Press, 1958.

Spowart, Andrew C. Teaching about alcohol abuse in a high school setting: A preventive or total abstinence approach? 1982. Educational Resources Information Center (ERIC) document number ED 225 046. (Microfiche)

Stainback, Robert D., and Rogers, Ronald W. Identifying effective components of alcohol abuse prevention programs: Effects of fear appeals, message style, and source expertise. *International Journal of the Addictions*, 1983, *18*, 393–405.

State Education Department of New York. *A Framework for Prevention.* Albany, NY: State Education Department, n.d.

Staulcup, Herbert J. Knowledge and Attitudes as Determinants of Alcohol Use Among Junior High School Students: Testing the Alcohol Education Assumption. Unpublished Ph.D. dissertation, Washington University, 1980.

Stehler, B. *The Alcohol Question in the Light of Social Ethics.* Westerville, OH: American Issue Press, 191–.

Stivers, Richard. Religion and Alcoholism. In: Kissin, Benjamin, and Begleiter, Henri (eds.) *The Pathogenesis of Alcoholism: Psychosocial Factors.* New York: Plenum, 1983. pp. 341–364.

Stolberg, Victor. Examination of the knowledge-attitudes-behavior model with incoming college students. *Journal of Alcohol and Drug Education*, 1987, *32*, 45–47.

Stover, Thomas R. An Attempt to Measure the Effects of a High School Alcohol Education Program. Unpublished M.S. thesis, University of Wisconsin at Stout, 1984.

Swisher, John D., Nesselroade, Cindy, and Tatanish, Coleen. Here's Looking at You Two is looking good: An experimental analysis. *Journal of Humanistic Education and Development*, 1985, *23*, 111–119.

Telfer, Elizabeth. Temperance. *Journal of Medical Ethics*, 1990, *16*, 157–159.

Terry, Theodore. An Evaluation of Alcohol Education in Grades Four, Five, and Six: An Analysis of Students' Self-Concept, Knowledge, Attitudes, and Decision-Making Skills. Unpublished Ph.D. dissertation, Brigham Young University, 1982.

Theurer, Karin L. Assessment of a Cognitive-Behavioral Alcohol Education Curriculum for the Prevention of Problem Drinking in Adolescents. Unpublished Ph.D. dissertation, State University of New York at Stony Brook, 1987.

Thompson, Merita L., Daugherty, Raymond, and Carter, Vivian. Alcohol education in schools: Toward a lifestyle risk-reduction approach. *Journal of School Health*, 1984, *54*, 79–83.

Thornton, Mark. *The Economics of Prohibition*. Salt Lake City, UT: University of Utah Press, 1991.

Tietsort, Francis J., (ed.) *Temperance—or Prohibition?* New York: American, 1929.

Timberlake, James H. *Prohibition and the Progressive Movement, 1900–1920*. Cambridge, MA: Harvard University Press, 1963.

Trefethen, Christine E. An Evaluation of the GAMES Alcohol Education Program. Unpublished M.A. thesis, Ball State University, 1993.

Tricker, Raymond. The Evolution and Documentation of the Implementation of Two Drug and Alcohol Curricula in Three Oregon School Districts. Unpublished Ph.D. dissertation, University of Oregon, 1985.

Tyack, David, B., and James, Thomas. Moral majorities and the school curriculum: Historical perspectives on the legalization of virtue. *Teachers College Record*, 1985, *86*, 513–537.

U.S. Congress. House. Title V, Drug-Free Schools and Communities Act of 1986. Sec. 5101–5192, Public Law 100–297. *United States Code*. 100th Cong., 2nd sess., 1988.

U.S. Department of Education. *Drug Prevention Curricula: A Guide to Selection and Implementation*. Washington, DC: U.S. Department of Education, 1988.

U.S. Department of Education. *What Works: Schools Without Drugs*. Washington, DC: U.S. Department of Education, 1992.

U.S. Department of Education. Office of Elementary and Secondary Education. Summary of Department of Education Drug Prevention Programs. Washington, DC: U.S. Department of Education. Office of Elementary and Secondary Education, January, 1993.

U.S. Department of Health and Human Services [DHEW]. *The Whole College Catalog About Drinking*. Washington, DC: National Institute on Alcoholism and Alcohol Abuse, 1976.

U.S. Department of Justice, Office of Justice Programs. *An Invitation to Project DARE: Drug Abuse Resistance Education*. Washington, DC: U.S. Department of Justice, 1988.

Unkovic, Charles M., Adler, Rudolf J., and Miller, Susan E. A Contemporary Study of Jewish Alcoholism—The Significant Other Point of View. In: Blaine, Allan (ed.) *Alcoholism and the Jewish Community*. New York: Federation of Jewish Philanthropies of New York, 1980. pp. 167–185.

Unterberger, Hilma, and DiCicco, Lena M. Alcohol education reevaluated. *Bulletin of the National Association of Secondary School Principals*, 1968, *52*, 15–29.

Upcraft, M. Lee, and Eck, William. TAPP: A Model Alcohol Education Program That Works. In: Goodale, Thomas G. (ed.) *Alcohol and the College Student*. San Francisco, CA: Jossey-Bass, 1986. pp. 35–41.

Wallack, Lawrence M. Mass media campaigns: The odds against finding behavior change. *Health Education Quarterly*, 1981, *8*, 209–260.

Warburton, Clark. *The Economic Results of Prohibition*. New York: Columbia University Press, 1932. Reprinted by AMS Press, New York, 1968.

Watts, Albert C. The Effectiveness of the School Health Curriculum in Preventing Cigarette Smoking and Alcohol Misuse: A Study of Behavior Intentions and Health Locus of Control. Unpublished Ph.D. dissertation, Virginia Commonwealth University, 1982.

Weisheit, Ralph A. The social context of alcohol and drug education: Implications for program evaluations. *Journal of Alcohol and Drug Education*, 1983, *29*, 72–81.

Weisheit, Ralph A., Hopkins, Ronald H., Kearney, Kathleen A., and Mauss, Armand L. The school as a setting for primary prevention. *Journal of Alcohol and Drug Education*, 1984, *30*, 27–35.

Whitehead, Paul C. Public policy and alcohol related damage: Media campaigns or social controls? *Addictive Behaviors*, 1979, *4*, 83–89.

Wiener, Carolyn. *The Politics of Alcoholism*. New Brunswick, NJ: Transaction Books, 1981.

Wilkinson, Rupert. *The Prevention of Drinking Problems: Alcohol Control and Cultural Influences*. New York, NY: Oxford University Press, 1970.

Willard, Frances. *Do Everything: A Handbook for the World's White Ribboners*. Chicago, IL: Gilbert, 1895.

Willebrandt, Mabel W. *The Inside of Prohibition*. Indianapolis, IN: Bobbs-Merrill, 1929.

Wilson, R., and Cordes, C. Congress votes to allow judges to strip federal aid from students convicted of using or selling drugs. *The Chronicle of Higher Education,* 1988 (November 2), A16, A25.

Wilusz, Janet, and Parker, Tommie L. Alcohol Education: A Study of High School Students' Knowledge and Attitude Toward Alcohol. Unpublished M.S.W. project, California State University at Sacramento, 1982.

Wodarski, John S. *The Role of Research in Clinical Practice*. Baltimore, MD: University Park Press, 1981.

Wodarski, John S. Evaluating a social learning approach to teaching adolescents about alcohol and driving: A multiple variable evaluation. *Journal of Social Service Research,* 1986–87, *30*, 27–35.

Wodarski, John S. A social learning approach to teaching adolescents about alcohol and driving: A multiple variable follow-up evaluation. *Journal of Behavior Therapy and Experimental Psychiatry*, 1987, *18*, 51–60.

Wodarski, John S., and Bordnick, Patrick S. Teaching adolescents about alcohol and driving: A 2-year follow-up study. *Research on Social Work Practice*, 1994, *4*, 28–39.

Wragg, Jeffrey. Drug and drug education: The development, design and longitudinal evaluation of an early childhood programme. *Australian Psychologist*, 1986, *21*, 283–298.

Yano, K., Rhoads, G. G., and Kagan, A. Coffee, alcohol and risk of coronary heart disease among Japanese men living in Hawaii. *New England Journal of Medicine*, 1977, *297*, 405–409.

Zeller, William J. Evaluating Alcohol Education Programming Strategies Within a University Residence Hall Environment. Unpublished Ph.D. dissertation, Iowa State University, 1985.

Ziegler, G. A., Rommell, W. E., and Herz, George. *Prohibition and Anti-Prohibition*. New York: Broadway Publishing Co., 1911.

Zimmer, Lynn, and Morgan, John P. Prohibition's Costs—Always Too High? Paper presented at the annual meetings of the Kettil Bruun Society for Social and Epidemiological Research on Alcohol. Toronto, Ontario, May 30–June 5, 1992.

Zimmerman, Jonathan. "The Queen of the Lobby": Mary Hunt, scientific temperance, and the dilemma of democratic education in America, 1879–1906. *History of Education Quarterly*, 1992, *32*, 1–30.

Zinberg, N. E. *Drug, Set, and Setting: The Basis for Controlled Intoxicant Use*. New Haven, CT: Yale University Press, 1984.

Zinberg, Norman E., and Fraser, Kathleen M. The Role of the Social Setting in the Prevention and Treatment of Alcoholism. In: Mendelson, Jack H., and Mello, Nancy K. (eds.) *The Diagnosis and Treatment of Alcoholism*. New York: McGraw-Hill, second edition, 1985. pp. 457–483.

Zuelke, Lisa K. The Effects of Drug Education on Alcohol Consumption. Unpublished M.A. thesis, Illinois State University, 1993.

Zylman, Richard. OVERemphasis on alcohol may be costing lives. *The Police Chief*, 1974, *41*, 64–67.

Subject Index

Author Index

About the Author

DAVID J. HANSON is Professor of Sociology at SUNY–Potsdam. A past president of the New York Sociological Association and recipient of the President's Award for Excellence in Research, he is the author of numerous works on alcohol and related subjects, including *Preventing Alcohol Abuse: Alcohol, Culture, and Control* (Praeger, 1995).

ISBN 0-275-95561-3

HARDCOVER BAR CODE